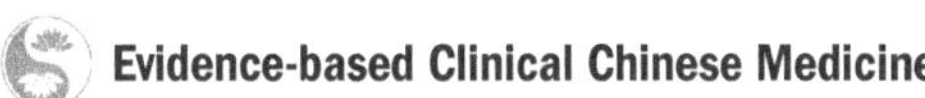
Evidence-based Clinical Chinese Medicine

Volume 16
Atopic Dermatitis

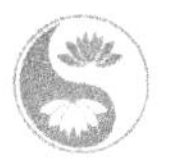 **Evidence-based Clinical Chinese Medicine**

Co Editors-in-Chief

Charlie Changli Xue
RMIT University, Australia

Chuanjian Lu
Guangdong Provincial Hospital of Chinese Medicine, China

Volume 16
Atopic Dermatitis

Lead Authors

Meaghan Coyle
RMIT University, Australia

Junfeng Liu
Guangdong Provincial Hospital of Chinese Medicine, China

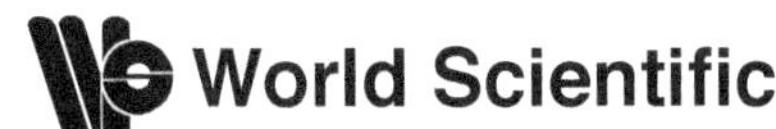 World Scientific

EW JERSEY • LONDON • SINGAPORE • BEIJING • SHANGHAI • HONG KONG • TAIPEI • CHENNAI • TOKYO

Published by

World Scientific Publishing Co. Pte. Ltd.

5 Toh Tuck Link, Singapore 596224

USA office: 27 Warren Street, Suite 401-402, Hackensack, NJ 07601

UK office: 57 Shelton Street, Covent Garden, London WC2H 9HE

Library of Congress Cataloging-in-Publication Data
Names: Xue, Charlie Changli, author. | Lu, Chuan-jian, 1964–   author.
Title: Evidence-based clinical Chinese medicine / Charlie Changli Xue, Chuanjian Lu.
Description: New Jersey : World Scientific, 2016. | Includes bibliographical references and index.
Identifiers: LCCN 2015030389| ISBN 9789814723084 (v. 1 : hardcover : alk. paper) |
    ISBN 9789814723091 (v. 1 : paperback : alk. paper) |
    ISBN 9789814723121 (v. 2 : hardcover : alk. paper) |
    ISBN 9789814723138 (v. 2 : paperback : alk. paper) |
    ISBN 9789814759045 (v. 3 : hardcover : alk. paper) |
    ISBN 9789814759052 (v. 3 : paperback : alk. paper)
Subjects: | MESH: Medicine, Chinese Traditional--methods. | Clinical Medicine--methods. |
    Evidence-Based Medicine--methods. | Psoriasis. | Pulmonary Disease, Chronic Obstructive.
Classification: LCC RC81 | NLM WB 55.C4 | DDC 616--dc23
LC record available at http://lccn.loc.gov/2015030389

Volume 16: Atopic Dermatitis
ISBN 978-981-120-611-5 (hardcover)
ISBN 978-981-123-541-2 (paperback)
ISBN 978-981-120-612-2 (ebook for institutions)
ISBN 978-981-120-613-9 (ebook for individuals)

First published 2020
Reprinted 2021

British Library Cataloguing-in-Publication Data
A catalogue record for this book is available from the British Library.

For any available supplementary material, please visit
https://www.worldscientific.com/worldscibooks/10.1142/11440#t=suppl

Disclaimer

The information in this book is based on systematic analyses of the best available evidence for Chinese medicine interventions both historical and contemporary. Every effort has been made to ensure accuracy and completeness of the data herein. This book is intended for clinicians, researchers and educators. The practice of evidence-based medicine consists of consideration of the best available evidence, practitioners' clinical experience and judgment, and patients' preference. Not all interventions are acceptable in all countries. It is important to note that some of the substances mentioned in this book may no longer be in use, may be toxic, or may be prohibited or restricted under the provisions of the Convention on International Trade in Endangered Species of Wild Fauna and Flora (CITES). Practitioners, researchers and educators are advised to comply with the relevant regulations in their country and with the restrictions on the trade in species included in CITES appendices I, II and III. This book is not intended as a guide for self-medication. Patients should seek professional advice from qualified Chinese medicine practitioners.

Foreword

Since the late 20th century, Chinese medicine, including acupuncture and herbal medicine, has been increasingly used throughout the world. The parallel development and spread of evidence-based medicine has provided challenges and opportunities for Chinese medicine. The opportunities have been evidence-based medicine's emphasis on the effective use of the best available clinical evidence, incorporating the clinicians' clinical experience, subject to patients' preference. Such practices have a patient focus which reflects the historical nature of Chinese medicine practice. However, the challenges are also significant due to the fact that, despite the long-term development and very rich literature accumulated over 2,000 years, there is an overall lack of high-level clinical evidence for many of the interventions used in Chinese medicine.

To address this knowledge gap, we need to generate clinical evidence through high-quality clinical studies and to evaluate evidence to enable effective use of such available evidence to promote evidence-based Chinese medicine practice.

Modern Chinese medicine is rooted in its classical literature and the legacies of ancient doctors, grounded in the practice of expert clinicians and increasingly informed by clinical and experimental research efforts. In recognition of the unique features of Chinese medicine, for each of the conditions in this series a 'whole-evidence' approach is used to provide a synthesis of different types and levels of evidence to enable practitioners to make clinical decisions informed by the current best evidence.

There are four main components of this 'whole-evidence' approach. In the first component, we present the current approaches to the diagnosis, differentiation and treatment of each condition based on expert consensus in published textbooks and clinical guidelines. This provides an overview of how the condition is currently managed. The second component provides an analysis of the condition in historical context based on systematic searches of the *Zhong Hua Yi Dian* which includes the full texts of more than 1,000 classical medical books. These analyses provide objective views on how the condition has been treated over two millennia, reveal continuities and discontinuities between traditional and modern practice, and suggest avenues for future research.

The third component is the assessment of evidence derived from modern clinical studies of Chinese medicine interventions. The methods established by the *Cochrane Collaboration* are used as the basis for conducting systematic reviews and undertaking meta-analyses of outcome data for randomised controlled trials (RCTs). In addition, the clinical relevance of meta-analysis data is enhanced by examining the herbal formulas, individual herbs and acupuncture treatments that were assessed in the RCTs, and the evidence base is broadened by the inclusion of data from controlled clinical trials and non-controlled studies. The fourth component is to determine how the herbal medicine interventions may achieve the effects indicated by the clinical trials. Thus for each of the most frequently used herbs we provide reviews of their effects in pre-clinical models and their likely mechanisms of action.

For each condition, this 'whole-evidence' approach links clinical expertise, historical precedent, clinical research data and experimental research to provide the reader with assessments of the current state of the evidence of efficacy and safety for Chinese medicine interventions using herbal medicines, acupuncture and moxibustion, and other health care practices such as *taichi*.

Since these books are available in Chinese and English, they can benefit patients, practitioners and educators internationally and enable practitioners to make clinical decisions informed by the current best evidence.

These publications represent a major milestone in Chinese medicine development and make a significant contribution to the evidence-based Chinese medicine development globally.

Co-Editors-in-Chief

Distinguished Professor Charlie Changli Xue, RMIT University, Australia

Professor Chuanjian Lu, Guangdong Provincial Hospital of Chinese Medicine, China

Purpose of this Book

This book is intended for clinicians, researchers and educators. It can be used to inform tertiary education and clinical practice by providing systematic, multidimensional assessments of the best available evidence for using Chinese medicine to manage each common clinical condition.

How to Use this Book

Some Definitions

A glossary is included, containing terms and definitions which frequently appear in the book. It also describes the definitions of statistical tests, methodological terms, evaluation tools and interventions. For example, in this book, integrative medicine refers to the combined use of a Chinese medicine treatment with conventional medical management, and combination therapies refer to two or more Chinese medicines from different therapy groups (e.g. Chinese herbal medicine, acupuncture or other Chinese medicine therapies) administered together. Terminology used throughout the monograph is based on the World Health Organisation's *Standard Terminologies on Traditional Medicine in the Western Pacific Region* (2007) where possible or from the cited reference.

Data Analysis and Interpretation of Results

In order to synthesise the clinical evidence, a range of statistical analysis approaches are used. In general, the effect size for dichotomous data is reported as a risk ratio (RR) with 95% confidence interval (CI), and for continuous data, they are reported as mean difference (MD) with 95% CI. Statistically significant effects are indicated with an asterisk*. Readers should note that statistical significance does not necessarily correspond with a clinically important effect. Interpretation of results should take into consideration the clinical significance, quality of studies (expressed as high, low or unclear risk of bias in this book) and heterogeneity amongst the studies. Tests for heterogeneity are conducted using the I^2 statistic. An I^2 score greater than 50% may indicate substantial heterogeneity.

Use of Evidence in Practice

The Grading of Recommendations Assessment, Development and Evaluation (GRADE) approach was used to summarise the quality of evidence and results of the strength of evidence for critical and important comparisons and outcomes. Due to the diverse nature of Chinese medicine practice, treatment recommendations are not included with the summary of findings tables. Therefore readers will need to interpret the evidence with reference to the local practice environment.

Limitations

Readers should note some of the methodological limitations on classical literature and clinical evidence.

- Search terms used to search the *Zhong Hua Yi Dian* database may not include all terms that have been used for the condition, which may alter the findings.
- Chinese language has changed over time. Citations have been interpreted for analysis, and such interpretations may be subject to disagreement.
- Chinese medicine theory has evolved over time. As such, concepts described in classical Chinese medical literature may no longer be found in contemporary works.

- Symptoms described in citations may be common to many conditions, and a judgment was required to determine the likelihood of the citation being related to the condition. This may have introduced some bias due to the subjective nature of the judgment.
- The vast majority of the clinical evidence for Chinese medicine treatments has come from China. The applicability of the findings to other populations and other countries requires further assessment.
- Many studies included participants with varying disease severity. Where possible, subgroup analyses were undertaken to examine the effects in different subpopulations. As this was not always possible, the findings may be limited to the population included, and not to subpopulations.
- The potential risk of bias found in many included studies suggested methodological limitations. The findings for GRADE assessments based on studies of very low to moderate quality evidence should be interpreted accordingly.
- Nine major English and Chinese language databases were searched to identify clinical studies, in addition to clinical trial registers. Other studies may exist which were not identified through searches, and which may alter the findings.
- The calculation of frequency of herbal formula use was based on formula names only. It is possible that studies evaluated herbal treatments with the same or similar herb ingredients, but which were given different formula names. Due to the complexity of herbal formulas, it was considered not appropriate to make a judgment as to the similarity of formulas for analysis. As such, the frequency of formulas reported in Chapter 5 may be underestimated.
- The most frequently utilised herbs which may have contributed to the treatment effect have been described in Chapter 5. These herbs may provide leads for further exploration. Calculation of the herbs with potential effect is based on frequency of formulas reported in the studies, and does not take into consideration the clinical implications and functions of every herb in a formula.

Authors and Contributors

Co-Editors-in-Chief

Prof. Charlie Changli Xue (*RMIT University, Australia*)
Prof. Chuanjian Lu (*Guangdong Provincial Hospital of Chinese Medicine, China*)

Co-Deputy Editors-in-Chief

Assoc. Prof. Anthony Lin Zhang (*RMIT University, Australia*)
Dr. Brian H May (*RMIT University, Australia*)
Prof. Xinfeng Guo (*Guangdong Provincial Hospital of Chinese Medicine, China*)
Prof. Zehuai Wen (*Guangdong Provincial Hospital of Chinese Medicine, China*)

Lead Authors

Dr. Meaghan Coyle (*RMIT University, Australia*)
Dr. Junfeng Liu (*Guangdong Provincial Hospital of Chinese Medicine, China*)

Co-Authors

RMIT University (Australia):
Assoc. Prof. Anthony Lin Zhang
Prof. Charlie Changli Xue

Guangdong Provincial Hospital of Chinese Medicine (China):

Prof. Chuanjian Lu
Prof. Xinfeng Guo
Prof. Hongyi Li
Dr. Xiumei Mo

Members of Advisory Committee and Panel

CO-CHAIRS OF PROJECT PLANNING COMMITTEE

Prof. Peter J Coloe (*RMIT University, Australia*)
Prof. Yubo Lyu (*Guangdong Provincial Hospital of Chinese Medicine, China*)
Prof. Dacan Chen (*Guangdong Provincial Hospital of Chinese Medicine, China*)

CENTRE ADVISORY COMMITTEE (IN ALPHABETICAL ORDER)

Prof. Keji Chen (*The Chinese Academy of Sciences, China*)
Prof. Aiping Lu (*Hong Kong Baptist University, China*)
Prof. Caroline Smith (*University of Western Sydney, Australia*)
Prof. David F Story (*RMIT University, Australia*)

METHODOLOGY EXPERT ADVISORY PANEL (IN ALPHABETICAL ORDER)

Prof. Zhaoxiang Bian (*Hong Kong Baptist University, China*)
Prof. Lixing Lao (*The University of Hong Kong, China*)
The late Prof. George Lewith (*University of Southampton, United Kingdom*)
Prof. Jianping Liu (*Beijing University of Chinese Medicine, China*)
Prof. Frank Thien (*Monash University, Australia*)
Prof. Jialiang Wang (*Sichuan University, China*)

CONTENT EXPERT ADVISORY PANEL (IN ALPHABETICAL ORDER)

Prof. Noel Cranswick (*The Royal Children's Hospital, Melbourne, Australia*)

Prof. Linfeng Li (*Beijing Friendship Hospital, Capital Medical University, China*)

Prof. Florian Pfab (*Technische Universität Munich, Germany*)

Prof. Liu Yang (*Southern Medical University, China*)

Distinguished Professor Charlie Changli Xue

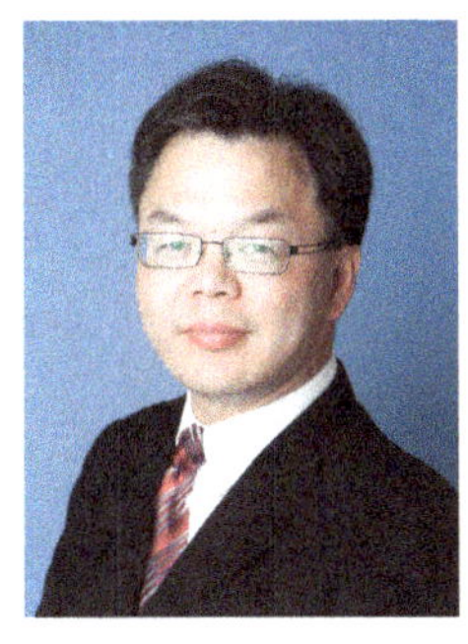

Professor Charlie Changli Xue holds a Bachelor of Medicine (majoring in Chinese Medicine) from Guangzhou University of Chinese Medicine, China (1987) and a PhD from RMIT University, Australia (2000). He has been an academic, researcher, regulator and practitioner for almost three decades. Professor Xue has made significant contributions to evidence-based educational development, clinical research, regulatory framework and policy development, and provision of high-quality clinical care to the community. Professor Xue is recognised internationally as an expert in evidence-based traditional medicine and integrative health care.

Professor Xue is the Inaugural National Chair of the Chinese Medicine Board of Australia appointed by the Australian Health Workforce Ministerial Council in 2011, and he was reappointed for a second term in 2014. Since 2007, he has been a Member of the World Health Organisation (WHO) Expert Advisory Panel for Traditional and Complementary Medicine, Geneva. Professor Xue is also Honorary Senior Principal Research Fellow at the Guangdong Provincial Academy of Chinese Medical Sciences, China.

At RMIT, Professor Xue is Executive Dean, School of Health and Biomedical Sciences. He is also Director of the WHO Collaborating Centre for Traditional Medicine.

Between 1995 and 2010, Professor Xue was Discipline Head of Chinese Medicine at RMIT University. He leads the development of five successful undergraduate and postgraduate degree programmes in Chinese Medicine at RMIT University which is now a global leader in Chinese medicine education and research.

Professor Xue's research has been supported by over AU$15 million research grants including six project grants from the Australian Government's National Health and Medical Research Council (NHMRC) and two Australian Research Council (ARC) grants. He has contributed over 200 publications and has been frequently invited as keynote speaker for numerous national and international conferences. Professor Xue has contributed to over 300 media interviews on issues related to complementary medicine education, research, regulation and practice.

Professor Chuanjian Lu

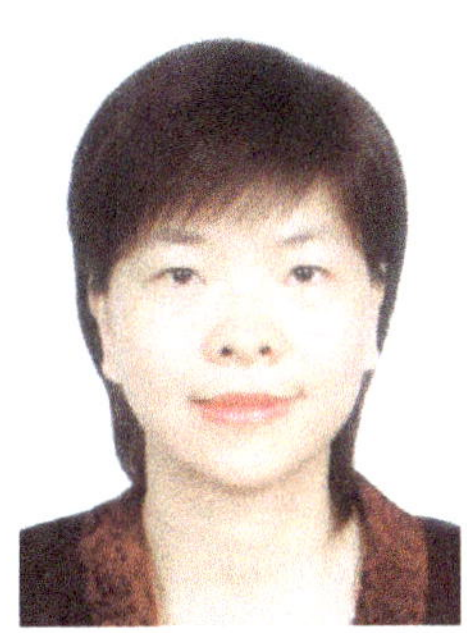

Professor Chuanjian Lu is the Vice-president of Guangdong Provincial Hospital of Chinese Medicine (Guangdong Provincial Academy of Chinese Medical Sciences, Second Clinical Medical College of Guangzhou University of Chinese Medicine). She is also the Chair of the Guangdong Traditional Chinese Medicine (TCM) Standardisation Technical Committee, and the Vice-chair of the Immunity Specialty Committee of the World Federation of Chinese Medicine Societies (WFCMS).

Professor Lu has engaged in scientific research into TCM, clinical practice and teaching for some 25 years. Her research has been devoted to integrating traditional and western medicine. She has edited and published 12 monographs and 120 academic research articles as first author and corresponding author with over 30 articles being included in SCI journals.

She has received widespread recognition for her achievements with awards for Excellent Teacher of South China, National Outstanding Women TCM Doctor, and National Outstanding Young Doctor of TCM. She also received the Science and Technology Star of the Association of Chinese Medicine, the National Excellent Science and Technology Workers of China Award and the Five-continent Women's Scientific Awards of China Medical Women's Association.

Professor Lu has won the Award of Science and Technology Progress over ten times from Guangdong Provincial Government, China Association of Chinese Medicine and Chinese Hospital Association.

Acknowledgements

The authors and contributors would like to acknowledge the valuable contributions of the following people who assisted with database searches, data extraction, data screening, data assessment, translation of documents, editing and/or administrative tasks: Jing Chen, Muyun Ding, Dr. Jhodie Duncan, Weiqiang Li, Yinzhe Lin, Dr. Shaonan Liu and Dr. Haiyan Wang.

Contents

List of Figures

List of Tables

1

Introduction to Atopic Dermatitis

OVERVIEW

Atopic dermatitis is a chronic skin condition which can occur in infants, children and adults. Skin lesions are typically accompanied by an itch, with lesion severity varying over time. Atopic dermatitis is a significant burden for patients and their family. Management options vary with lesion severity, ranging from skin care to systemic immunomodulatory therapy. Patient education is important to improve symptoms, reduce relapse and improve quality of life.

Definition of Atopic Dermatitis

Atopic dermatitis is a chronic inflammatory skin condition which typically starts during childhood and may persist into adulthood.[1] Skin lesions are often accompanied by an itch (pruritus), which contributes to the burden associated with atopic dermatitis. The clinical course is characterised by periods of exacerbation and remission.[2]

The term 'eczema' is used as an umbrella term to describe inflammatory skin diseases, of which the most common is atopic dermatitis. Other eczema conditions include seborrheic dermatitis and contact dermatitis.[3] 'Atopy' refers to the genetic tendency to develop allergic conditions such as allergic rhinitis and allergic asthma, and is associated with heightened immune response to common allergens.[4] Atopic dermatitis is synonymous with atopic eczema.[1,5]

Clinical Presentation and Subtypes of Atopic Dermatitis

The characteristic signs of atopic dermatitis include erythema, dry skin (xerosis), excoriation, weeping/oozing and crusting (exudation), and skin thickening (lichenification).[1] In the acute stage, erythema is poorly defined and skin surface changes may include excoriation, exudation, crusting or scaling.[6,7] Chronic lesions present with infiltrated erythema, lichenification, prurigo, crusts and scales.[6] Lichenification is caused by chronic inflammation, often due to repeated scratching and rubbing.[7] Dry skin may be present in the absence of active skin lesions.[7] Pruritus may be present during the day and is usually worse at night.[8] Throughout the clinical course, atopic dermatitis lesions tend to recur at the same sites.[9] The local molecular and/or cellular changes persist after clinical resolution of atopic dermatitis lesions, predisposing the area to future flare-ups.[10]

Werfel *et al.* (2014)[11] suggest that clinical presentation of atopic dermatitis varies according to age and stage (acute or chronic). Infants may present with scalp dermatitis ('cradle cap') or generalised disease, which usually spares the groin/nappy area.[11] Infants and children may have involvement of the head, neck, and extensor surfaces of arms and legs.[1] Children, adolescents and adults typically have flexural dermatitis on the elbow (antecubital fossa) and back of the knee (popliteal fossa).[1] In adolescents and adults, dermatitis may present on the hand, while Besnier prurigo (prurigo associated with dermatitis) are intensely itchy spots that can be found on the shoulder and arms in adults.[11] Besnier prurigo can be either papular or nodular.

Even within different ages, clinical diversity may exist. A Korean study of 5,000 patients diagnosed with atopic dermatitis, most of whom were adults, found that 89% presented with typical age-based distribution.[12] The main sites of atopic dermatitis were the neck and head for infants and adults, and the upper extremities were the most affected part in children aged two to 12. Atopic dermatitis lesions were found throughout the body in 46% of patients, followed by the head/neck (35%), upper extremities (33%), lower extremities (25%)

and trunk (16%). All atopic dermatitis patients reported pruritus. In a community-based survey of Singaporeans, flexural involvement was more common (cubital fossa 51.7%; popliteal fossa 41.6%).[13]

Atopic dermatitis can be categorised as either extrinsic or intrinsic. In extrinsic atopic dermatitis, immunoglobulin (Ig) E is elevated and there is a history of atopic disease. Intrinsic, or non-allergic, atopic dermatitis presents with lesions in the absence of increased IgE and atopic disease. Extrinsic cases with elevated IgE are more common than intrinsic atopic dermatitis.[14]

Epidemiology

Diversity in nomenclature and diagnostic criteria for atopic dermatitis over time have complicated estimates of prevalence and incidence.[15,16] The International Study of Asthma and Allergies in Childhood (ISAAC) used a standardised definition to assess the prevalence of atopic diseases including eczema in 56 countries.[17] The first phase of the study, involving more than 256,000 children, found that prevalence was higher in Northern Europe and Australasia, and lower in Eastern Europe, Central Europe and Asia.[17] Eczema was estimated to affect between 5% and 20% of children aged six to seven and 13 to 14 years.

In the third phase of the ISAAC study, involving over one million children in 60 countries, prevalence ranged from 0.9% (India) to 22.5% (Ecuador) in six- to seven-year-olds, and from 0.2% (China) to 24.6% (Columbia) in 13- to 14-year-olds.[18] Eczema prevalence was lower for boys than girls. Changes in prevalence between phases one and three of the study were generally small.[19] An increase in prevalence was seen in children aged six to seven years, while mixed results were seen for 13- to 14-year-old children, with some decreases in developed countries and some increases in developing countries.[19] Eczema prevalence for a period of 12 months among six- to seven-year-olds in Melbourne, Australia was 17.1% in phase three of the study,[20] rising from 11.1% in phase one. Little change was seen in prevalence among 13- to 14-year-olds in China between phases one (1.2%) and three (1.4%).[20]

Several studies have reported on the prevalence of atopic dermatitis in Chinese populations.[21–23] Prevalence from a cross-sectional study of dermatology outpatients (including both adults and children) was found to be 7.8%.[22] A subset of data from the same study found lower prevalence in adults (4.6%).[23] Geographic location was shown to be a factor in the Chinese study, with higher prevalence at latitudes of 25–30°N than other latitudes. Point-prevalence in children aged one to seven years based on clinical diagnosis was 13%, and when diagnosis was made according to the United Kingdom Working Party's diagnostic criteria, prevalence was lower (4.8%).[21] Data from the United States (US) 2003 National Survey of Children's Health found that 10.7% of children were diagnosed with eczema in the previous month.[24] Prevalence ranged from 8.7% to 18.1% across states, with higher prevalence seen in urban areas, among African Americans and in households with tertiary education.

Burden

Atopic dermatitis has significant physical, psychological and financial burdens. Of all skin disorders included in the Global Burden of Disease Study 2010, eczema had the highest number of disability-adjusted life years.[25] Health-related quality of life has been demonstrated to decrease as severity of atopic dermatitis increases;[16] although even mild symptoms can cause significant emotional distress in patients.[11] The burden from physical symptoms is considerable. Despite the use of systemic therapies, more than 50% of 380 patients in a clinical trial reported problematic itch frequency and atopic dermatitis-related sleep disturbances.[26] In addition to itch and sleep disturbance, children experience burden due to treatment, impact on social activities such as sport, and embarrassment from their eczema.[27]

Atopic dermatitis also has an impact on psychological well-being. Parents reported emotional problems in their children, including crying, irritability, behavioural problems and problems associated with treatment.[28] The US National Health and Wellness Survey of adults over 18 years of age found people with atopic dermatitis (n = 428) were younger and consisted of a higher proportion of females than people without atopic dermatitis (n = 74,752).[29] Further, the cohort with atopic dermatitis had higher prevalence of other atopic and neuropsychiatric diseases such as anxiety and depression.

The burden from atopic dermatitis is also experienced by parents, other caregivers and the family. Chernyshov (2016)[30] described how the burden of atopic dermatitis changes as the child grows. Parental exhaustion of children aged up to three years can lead to exacerbation of symptoms and psychological changes in the child. Children aged between three and ten may experience bullying, teasing or exclusion, and older children can be more self-critical and have lower self-esteem. A qualitative study found having a child with atopic dermatitis increased the physical burden for parents, with extra requirements for washing, cleaning and shopping.[31] Children's sleep disturbance also disrupted the sleep of parents, and tiredness limited the parents' social life. The additional burden for parents left them feeling exhausted, anxious, guilty, resentful, frustrated and/or helpless.

The financial burden of atopic dermatitis includes both direct costs such as medical fees, medication/over-the-counter treatments, diet or clothing requirements, and indirect costs such as pain, suffering and absenteeism.[32] A conservative estimate from 2015 of the annual costs associated with atopic dermatitis in the United States was 5.297 billion US dollars; actual cost is likely to be higher due to increased prevalence over time.[27] Health care resource utilisation has been shown to be higher in patients with atopic dermatitis than in matched controls without atopic dermatitis.[33] Expenses for health service utilisation were twice as high among people with atopic dermatitis than those without the disease.[29] Out-of-pocket expenses for health service utilisation due to atopic dermatitis was 489 USD per person per year.[34] Inpatient costs for atopic dermatitis in the United States were 127.8 million USD, with inpatient costs greater for adults than for children (8.3 million USD compared to 3.3 million USD, respectively).[35] Average annual out-of-pocket expenses in Australia was 425 AU dollars per person per year.[36]

The indirect costs of atopic dermatitis have been found to be substantially more than the direct costs.[32] Absenteeism contributed to indirect costs, with 2.3% of people surveyed by Silverberg (2015)[34] missing three or more days of work due to eczema. Atopic dermatitis may also impact on career progression.[37] Both Whiteley *et al.* (2016)[29] and Eckert *et al.* (2017)[33] posit that the significant burden experienced by people with atopic dermatitis suggests 'an unmet need for more effective management strategies'.[29]

Risk Factors

Family history of atopic disease is an important risk factor.[1,12] Filaggrin (FLG) gene mutations confer a specific risk for atopic dermatitis.[1] Products of FLG degradation are components of natural moisturising factors which contribute to maintaining skin barrier function.[1] A review of the epidemiology of childhood atopic dermatitis highlights a positive correlation with latitude and a negative correlation with annual outdoor temperature.[38] Other risk factors identified from the review include a 'western' diet, obesity, low levels of physical activity, reduced diversity in bacterial gut flora and prior use of broad spectrum antibiotics. Risk factors identified among Chinese children included passive smoke exposure, premature birth and fussy food preferences.[21] Environmental risk factors identified in a review by Kantor and Silverberg (2017)[39] include prenatal exposure to stress, antibiotics and alcohol. Other potential risk factors identified in the American Academy of Dermatology's 2014 guidelines[1] include being African-American, parents having a higher education level, and living in urban areas.

Protective factors identified in the review by Flohr and Mann (2014)[38] support the 'hygiene hypothesis.' This includes helminth infection during pregnancy, maternal contact with farm animals during pregnancy, and early-life exposure to dogs and high-level endotoxins.[38] Other protective factors highlighted by Kantor and Silverberg[39] included early day care, and consumption of unpasteurised milk, omega-3 long chain fatty acids and probiotics. Living in a rural area and older age were protective factors among Chinese children.[21] In comparison, several factors have been identified which may aggravate atopic dermatitis. These include exposure to irritants, pruritogens, air pollution or tobacco smoke,[39] hot weather/dry weather/seasonal changes,[12,13] exposure to dusty environments,[13] physical exercise[13] and stress.[12]

Pathological Processes

Atopic dermatitis is a multifactorial disease arising from a combination of genetic and environmental factors, immune dysfunction, skin barrier defects and increased skin infections.[9] The relative contribution of each is not yet understood.[9] As described above, one of the most significant genetic factors in the development of atopic dermatitis is a loss of function mutation in the FLG gene.[40,41] Filaggrin is involved in keratinocyte development, contributes to the formation of corneocytes for the stratum corneum (SC) and aggregates the keratin cytoskeleton.[41,42] Degradation products of filaggrin contribute to the natural moisturising factor and maintaining skin pH, thus maintaining integrity of the skin barrier.[43] Loss of function mutations of the FLG gene contribute to increased skin pH, impaired skin integrity and decreased hydration.[9] Other genetic factors important to atopy and inflammation, such as mutations of the serine peptidase inhibitor Kazal type 5 (SPINK5) gene, have been highlighted by Mao *et al.* (2014).[40]

Gene-environment interactions have also been suggested as contributing to the development of atopic diseases, particularly in early life. Exposure to cats (but not dogs) in early life has been shown to increase the risk of developing atopic dermatitis in children with FLG loss of function variants.[44] As children in this study had not developed cat-specific IgE antibodies, the mechanism was deemed not related to allergy. In Korean children with a parental history of atopy, moving into a newly built home in the first year of life was associated with an increased risk of developing atopic dermatitis.[45] Conversely, a twin population study from Germany found that early-life risk factors did not modify the genetic influence on development of atopic dermatitis.[46]

The 'inside-out' hypothesis suggests that atopic dermatitis is cytokine driven, resulting in reactive epidermal hyperplasia.[9] The immune response in atopic dermatitis presents with two distinct phases. The initial and acute phase is characterised by a predominant T helper cell type 2 (Th2) response, with increased levels of interleukin (IL)-4, IL-5, IL-13, thymic stromal lymphopoietin (TSLP) and eosinophils.[40,41] These changes have been found in both lesional and non-lesional skin.[40] Damaged keratinocytes trigger inflammation through TSLP.[39] Thymic stromal lymphopoietin, in concert with IL-25 and IL-33, is involved in activating the Th2 response seen in both the acute and chronic phase of atopic dermatitis.[9,41,43,47] The cytokines IL-4 and IL-13 released from Th2 cells are considered to promote IgE production and atopy,[47,48] and suppress antimicrobial peptide (AMP) production.[39] Cytokines IL-4 and IL-13 contribute to inflammation,[43] and IL-31 inhibits epidermal differentiation and induces pruritus.[43]

In the chronic phase, higher levels of interferon (IFN)-γ, IL-5, IL-12 and granulocyte-macrophage colony stimulating factor (GM-CSF) indicate Th1 dominance.[40,41] T helper cell type 1 secretes IFN-γ to kill intracellular pathogens whilst suppressing Th2-mediated immunity.[47] Interleukin-5 and IL-12 support the development of eosinophils and macrophages, and promote Th1 inflammation.[48] Expression of Th1 cytokines is not detected in acute skin lesions.[40] T helper cell type 22 and Th17 have also been implicated in the chronic phase of atopic dermatitis.[49] T helper cell type 22 releases cytokine IL-22 which has been shown to down-regulate skin barrier function.[9] Thymic stromal lymphopoietin, IL4, and to a lesser extent IL-13, IL-17, IL-22 and IL31, can also induce acquired reduction in filaggrin function.[47] T helper cell type 17 secretes proinflammatory cytokine IL-17 which mediates inflammation and autoimmunity.[43]

Regulatory T cells (Tregs) contribute to the control of allergic responses through suppressing immunity[50] and promoting homeostasis.[51] Research suggests that increased Tregs in early life may be protective against allergies.[50] The role of Tregs in allergic outcomes in the first year of life was examined using the biomarker transcription factor Forkhead/winged-helix transcription factor box P3 (Foxp3).[52] Children born with lower numbers of cord blood Tregs were at a significantly higher risk of developing atopic dermatitis in the first year of life. Genetic and environmental factors were seen to influence developmental of Tregs *in utero*. The frequency of another Treg biomarker, CD25[hi] T cells, has been found to be higher in people with atopic dermatitis compared to controls with low total levels of IgE.[53] In the same study, CD25[hi] T cell levels were shown to decrease as skin condition improved in three patients with severe disease, suggesting Treg involvement in atopic dermatitis.

Skin barrier dysfunction also plays a role in the development of atopic dermatitis. This is described as the 'outside-in' hypothesis.[9] The outer layer of the skin, the SC, is composed of proteins such as FLG, loricin and involucrin, and a lipid layer of long-chain ceramides, cholesterol and free fatty acids.[43] The SC protects the body against allergens, microbial infection, irritant, and physical changes, and prevents water loss through the skin (trans-epidermal water loss, TEWL).[43] The SC is composed of anucleated corneocytes[54] which secrete substances such as FLG. These substances break down, producing amino acids that contribute to the natural moisturising factor and lipids, such as ceramides, that contribute to the structure and water-holding capacity of the skin.[47]

In patients with atopic dermatitis the lipid layer is altered, with decreased levels of ceramides and increased levels of short-chain fatty acids.[43] The altered levels of ceramides and short-chain fatty acids lead to abnormal lipid organisation[43] which is associated with atopic dermatitis severity regardless of mutations in the FLG gene.[55] Furthermore, increased levels of short-chain fatty acids were found in unaffected (non-lesional) skin of patients with atopic dermatitis,[55] highlighting that skin barrier alterations can be found in both affected and unaffected skin.[47]

Keratinocytes, found in the basal layer of the skin, perform several key roles. Keratinocytes generate AMPs, which clear pathogens and maintain the epidermal layer as part of innate immunity.[43] Antimicrobial peptides bind to the cell walls of pathogens to promote cell lysis, and produce cytokines and chemokines to recruit neutrophils, monocytes, mast cells and T cells.[43] The main classes of skin AMPs are cathelicidin and human β-defensins 2 and 3. Both are found to be reduced in atopic dermatitis, leaving patients prone to bacterial and viral infections.[43] The reduction in AMPs may not be a result of a defect in epidermal cells, but rather mediated by cytokines produced by infiltrating cells.[48] In addition, FLG deficiency may impair AMP function.[9]

Colonisation of the lesional and non-lesional skin with *Staphylococcus aureus* is common in people with atopic dermatitis.[54] This is due to both an impaired skin barrier and impaired immune responses.[56] *Staphylococcus aureus* decreases the integrity of the skin barrier through protease activity, activates eosinophils and basophils, and induces toxin-specific IgE secretion.[9,57] *Staphylococcus aureus* can aggravate, or exacerbate, skin lesions.[58] Other pathogens found to inhabit the skin microbiome in people with atopic dermatitis include *Malassezia furfur* and *Candida albicans*.[57] Other aggravators include environmental factors such as dust mites and soap, mechanical trauma and scratching.[41]

Diagnosis

Diagnosis of atopic dermatitis is based on clinical presentation and patient/family history.[1] Several criteria have been developed to aid diagnosis, and there is no 'gold standard'.[59] Two of the most commonly used are the Hanifin and Rajka criteria,[60] and the United Kingdom (UK) Working Party.[61] The criteria proposed by Hanifin and Rajka require at least three of the four major features and at least three of 23 minor features. Major features include pruritus, typical presentation of eczema (morphology and distribution), chronic/relapsing course and personal/family medical history; minor features include symptoms such as xerosis, early age of onset and elevated serum IgE. The UK Working Party revised the Hanifin and Rajka criteria, with one major criteria (itchy skin condition, or parent report of scratching or rubbing by a child), and three or more additional features required for a diagnosis of atopic dermatitis.[62] Minor features include history of flexural involvement, personal history of asthma or hay fever, history of generally dry skin, visible flexural eczema and onset under the age of two.[62]

Guidelines of the American Academy of Dermatology (AAD)[1] and the Japanese Society of Allergology[6] no longer require early onset as an essential criterion for diagnosis. The AAD proposed that essential features include pruritus and eczema with typical morphology and chronic/relapsing history, age, xerosis and history of atopy such as personal/family history or IgE reactivity. The European consensus-based (S2k) guideline[5] recommends examination of the entire skin organ for diagnosis.

Laboratory tests are not recommended for diagnosis or assessment of disease severity as no reliable tests can distinguish atopic dermatitis from other diseases.[1] Serum IgE may, or may not, be elevated in people with atopic dermatitis, and this test is not recommended as a diagnostic tool or as a reliable marker of disease severity.[1] Serum IgE, skin biopsy, genetic testing and/or patch testing may be used to exclude other pathologies.[1] Diagnosis also requires exclusion of other skin conditions such as seborrheic dermatitis, contact dermatitis, scabies, psoriasis, irritant/toxic contact eczema, microbial eczema, cutaneous T-cell lymphoma, photosensitivity dermatoses, ichthyoses, erythroderma due to other causes and immune deficiency diseases associated with eczema.[1,11] In infants, seborrheic dermatitis and atopic dermatitis may overlap. Seborrheic dermatitis usually presents without pruritus and may appear anywhere on the body, while atopic dermatitis usually spares the groin/nappy area.[1]

Complications of atopic dermatitis include viral or fungal infections, and secondary bacterial infections.[5] Rare complications include eye diseases, growth delay and alopecia areata.[5] Other infections observed during treatment with topical calcineurin inhibitors (TCI) include eczema herpeticum and eczema molluscatum.[63]

Management

Nine clinical practice guidelines were identified for atopic dermatitis and were reviewed to guide the content hereafter. Two guidelines were from the US:

- The guidelines of the American Academy of Dermatology (AAD).[1,64–66]

- The Joint Task Force on Practice Parameters (JTFPP) 2012,[8] representing the American Academy of Allergy, Asthma and Immunology, the American College of Allergy, Asthma and Immunology, and the Joint Council of Allergy, Asthma and Immunology.

Two guidelines were from Europe:

- The European consensus-based (S2k) guideline.[5]
- The European Task Force on Atopic Dermatitis/EADV Eczema Task Force position paper 2015.[67]

Two guidelines were from Japan:

- The Japanese Society of Allergology.[6]
- The Japanese Dermatology Association.[68]

Other guidelines from the Asia-Pacific region included the Chinese Society of Dermatology guideline;[69] the Consensus Guidelines for the Treatment of Atopic Dermatitis in Korea[63,70] and the Asia-Pacific consensus guidelines.[71] The key guideline recommended treatments are summarised in Table 1.1.

As atopic dermatitis is a chronic condition, treatment involves a long-term management plan.[67] Treatment goals are to prevent complications, control symptoms, reduce the severity and extent of disease, prevent or reduce remission, and improve quality of life.[71] This is achieved through a combination of strategies, including ensuring adequate skin hydration, the use of anti-inflammatory and antipruritic therapies, and avoiding exacerbating factors.[8] A stepped care approach is described in the guidelines, with many recommending treatments based on atopic eczema severity.[5,6,8,67,68]

Basic therapy includes emollients/moisturisers, skin cleansing, bath additives (for the last two minutes of bathing), education and avoidance of irritants/aggravating factors.[8,67] Maintaining adequate skin hydration is achieved through the use of emollients or moisturisers, which are most beneficial when applied after bathing when the skin is moist.[64] Emollients can be expensive considering the volume

Table 1.1. Summary of Recommended Treatments in Clinical Guidelines

Severity	Treatment
No lesions/dry skin	Skin care, patient education, identification/avoidance of triggers.
Mild	Skin care, patient education, identification/avoidance of triggers; plus topical corticosteroids/topical glucocorticoids, and/or topical calcineurin inhibitors e.g. pimecrolimus, tacrolimus.
Moderate	Skin care, patient education, identification/avoidance of triggers; plus stronger topical steroids and/or topical calcineurin inhibitors.
Severe	Skin care, patient education, identification/avoidance of triggers; plus systemic immunomodulatory therapy e.g. cyclosporine A, azathioprine, methotrexate, mycophenolate mofetil, interferon gamma and/or short-term use of systemic steroids.
Other Treatments	
Adjunctive agents	Oral antihistamines, identification/avoidance of triggers and psychosomatic/psychological interventions.
Therapy for complications	Oral and/or topical antibiotics and antiviral drugs for bacterial/viral infections.
Non-pharmacological	Phototherapy.

Adapted from Eichenfield *et al.* (2014),[64] Katayama *et al.* (2017),[6] Saeki *et al.* (2016),[68] Schneider *et al.* (2013),[8] Sidbury *et al.* (2014),[65] Sidbury *et al.* (2014)[66] and Werfel *et al.* (2016).[5]

required for entire skin coverage, while moisturisers containing glycerol or 5% urea (if tolerated) can be applied twice daily.[67] Moisturising the skin can reduce pruritus.[68]

Skin cleansers should be non-irritant and low allergenic, with pH between 5 and 6.[67] Bathing is important for skin hydration and to wash away irritants such as sweat,[6] bacteria in cases of infection[67] and other irritants. Warm baths for at least ten minutes can aid hydration.[8] Education is important to improve treatment adherence and self-management.[67] Education programmes may involve dermatologists, paediatricians, dietitians, nurses and psychologists, and have been shown to be beneficial.[66,67] Parental education is important for successful management of atopic dermatitis in children.[72] Irritants and allergens vary, and may include clothing, food allergies, furred pets (particularly cats), pollen and indoor aeroallergens.[67] Guidelines vary in their recommendations regarding irritants and allergens, with some supporting strategies such as silver-impregnated or silk clothes and antimicrobial underwear,[5,67] minimising exposure to aeroallergens[8] and environmental modifications,[8] while others suggest there is lack of evidence for these strategies.[73]

Pharmacological Treatments

Pharmacologic treatment of atopic dermatitis is predominantly through topical therapies used alone or in combination with systemic agents, or other therapies such as phototherapy.[64]

Topical Therapies

Guidelines recommend the use of topical corticosteroids (TCS) and TCI for treatment of flares and for maintenance/proactive therapy. Topical corticosteroids have anti-inflammatory, vasoconstrictive and immunosuppressive actions,[71] and act on a range of immune cells to inhibit release of proinflammatory cytokines.[64] These vary in strength, and should be selected according to severity, location and patient age.[5,71] Topical corticosteroids should be applied once or twice daily to treat flare-ups until under control.[64,71] There is no standard dose to be used for flare-ups.[64] Care should be taken when applying corticosteroids to areas of thin skin where greater absorption is likely.[64] Topical calcineurin inhibitors are anti-inflammatory drugs which also have an immunomodulatory action.[64,71] Topical calcineurin inhibitors act through inhibiting T cell activation, disrupting production of proinflammatory cytokines and other mediators of inflammatory reactions.[64] The two TCIs currently used for atopic dermatitis are pimecrolimus and tacrolimus.

Proactive therapy involves long-term intermittent use of anti-inflammatory therapy (usually twice weekly) to areas where lesions typically appear with emollient applied to the entire skin.[9,67]

Proactive/maintenance therapy may use TCS, TCI or a combination of both.[6] For long-term management, the lowest strength of corticosteroid that is effective should be used.[64]

Systemic Agents

When disease control with topical therapies is inadequate or not achieved, or where disease is persistent and widespread, systemic agents may be considered.[65,71] Systemic immunomodulatory agents include cyclosporine A, azathioprine, methotrexate, mycophenolate mofetil and IFN-γ.[65] In cases of infection, oral and/or topical antibiotics or antiviral/antifungal treatments should be applied.[68] There is disagreement across guidelines as to whether topical antiseptics should be used although bleach baths are often recommended.[74] Antihistamines and antiallergenic treatments may be helpful to reduce pruritus in some patients.[8] When sleep is disturbed, sedating first-generation antihistamines may be considered.[73] Topical antihistamines are not recommended.[64]

Non-pharmacological Treatments

Phototherapy should be considered as second-line therapy after failure of first-line treatment with emollients, TCS and/or TCI.[65] Types of phototherapy include natural sunlight, narrow band (NB) ultraviolet (UV)B, broad band (BB) UVB, UVA, topical and systemic psoralen plus UVA (PUVA), UVA and B (UVAB), and Goeckerman therapy (use of crude coal tar with UV light).[65] Some guidelines recommend restrictions based on age. The Asia-Pacific and S2k guidelines recommend phototherapy be reserved for adults and children over 12 years of age.[5,71] The use of laser therapy is not recommended.[65]

Wet wrap therapy is recommended for significant lesions.[64] In wet wrap therapy, a topical agent is applied to the lesion. This is then covered by a wet first layer of dressing followed by a dry outer layer. This approach increases penetration of the topical agent, provides a barrier against scratching and decreases water loss.[64] Wet wraps can be left *in situ* for up to 24 hours, and can be applied at home or during hospitalisation.

Psychosomatic and/or psychological care may be considered for patients suffering psychological distress and for those whose distress affects their treatment adherence.[5,6,8,68] Various other treatments are described in the guidelines, with varying amounts and levels of evidence, and a lack of consensus across guidelines. These include antipruritic agents i.e., shale oil and coal tar,[5,67] zinc,[5] bleach baths used to decolonise *Staphylococcus aureus*,[8,64,71] climate therapy,[67] immunotherapy[5] and n-3 polyunsaturated fatty acid.[6]

Several of the reviewed guidelines included evaluation of evidence for complementary and alternative medicines (CAM). Most guidelines which included CAM concluded that there is insufficient evidence to support their use for atopic dermatitis, and their use should be reviewed when further controlled studies are available.[5] The use of Chinese herbal medicine (CHM) is common in many Asian countries, and this is reflected in clinical guidelines. The guidelines of the Japanese Dermatology Association recommend CHM as combination therapy where inadequate response has been achieved with topical anti-inflammatory agents, skin care and trigger avoidance strategies.[68] The Japanese Society of Allergology also supports the use of some CHMs with proven efficacy.[6] The Korean consensus guidelines acknowledge that Korean herbal medicine use is common; however, the evidence remains insufficient to recommend its use, and safety remains a concern.[70]

Prognosis

Many children with atopic dermatitis have resolution before adulthood, although between 10% and 30% continue to experience symptoms into adulthood.[75] With adequate management, the intervals between relapse can be extended, and the burden experienced by patients can be reduced.[6] Patient education should be emphasised at each consultation, including treatment doses, stepping up or down treatment, infection and skin care advice which is culturally appropriate.[71]

References

1. Eichenfield LF, Tom WL, Chamlin SL, *et al.* (2014) Guidelines of care for the management of atopic dermatitis: Section 1. Diagnosis and assessment of atopic dermatitis. *J Am Acad Dermatol* **70**(2): 338–351.
2. Katayama I, Kohno Y, Akiyama K, *et al.* (2014) Japanese guideline for atopic dermatitis 2014. *Allergol Int* **63**(3): 377–398.
3. Silvestre Salvador JF, Romero-Perez D, Encabo-Duran B. (2017) Atopic dermatitis in adults: A diagnostic challenge. *J Investig Allergol Clin Immunol* **27**(2): 78–88.
4. American Academy of Allergy Asthma & Immunology. (2017) Atopy. Available from: https://www.aaaai.org/conditions-and-treatments/conditions-dictionary/atopy.
5. Werfel T, Heratizadeh A, Aberer W, *et al.* (2016) S2k guideline on diagnosis and treatment of atopic dermatitis: Short version. *Allergo J Int* **25**: 82–95.
6. Katayama I, Aihara M, Ohya Y, *et al.* (2017) Japanese guidelines for atopic dermatitis 2017. *Allergol Int* **66**(2): 230–247.
7. Rycroft RJG, Robertson SJ, Wakelin SH. (2010) *Dermatology: A Colour Handbook*, 2nd ed. Manson Publishing, London.
8. Schneider L, Tilles S, Lio P, *et al.* (2013) Atopic dermatitis: A practice parameter update 2012. *J Allergy Clin Immunol* **131**(2): 295–299. e1–e27.
9. Czarnowicki T, Krueger JG, Guttman-Yassky E. (2014) Skin barrier and immune dysregulation in atopic dermatitis: An evolving story with important clinical implications. *J Allergy Clin Immunol Pract* **2**(4): 371–379; quiz 80–81.
10. Suarez-Farinas M, Gittler JK, Shemer A, *et al.* (2013) Residual genomic signature of atopic dermatitis despite clinical resolution with narrowband UVB. *J Allergy Clin Immunol* **131**(2): 577–579.
11. Werfel T, Schwerk N, Hansen G, *et al.* (2014) The diagnosis and graded therapy of atopic dermatitis. *Dtsch Arztebl Int* **111**(29–30): 509–520, i.
12. Chu H, Shin JU, Park CO, *et al.* (2017) Clinical diversity of atopic dermatitis: A review of 5,000 patients at a single institute. *Allergy Asthma Immunol Res* **9**(2): 158–168.
13. Cheok S, Yee F, Ma JYS, *et al.* (2018) Prevalence and descriptive epidemiology of atopic dermatitis and its impact on quality of life in Singapore. *Br J Dermatol* **178**(1): 276–277.

14. Wuthrich B, Schmid-Grendelmeier P. (2003) The atopic eczema/dermatitis syndrome. Epidemiology, natural course, and immunology of the IgE-associated ("extrinsic") and the nonallergic ("intrinsic") AEDS. *J Investig Allergol Clin Immunol* **13**(1): 1–5.

15. Deckers IA, McLean S, Linssen S, *et al.* (2012) Investigating international time trends in the incidence and prevalence of atopic eczema 1990–2010: A systematic review of epidemiological studies. *PLoS One* **7**(7): e39803.

16. Silverberg JI. (2017) Public health burden and epidemiology of atopic dermatitis. *Dermatol Clin* **35**(3): 283–289.

17. Williams H, Robertson C, Stewart A, *et al.* (1999) Worldwide variations in the prevalence of symptoms of atopic eczema in the International Study of Asthma and Allergies in Childhood. *J Allergy Clin Immunol* **103**(1 Pt 1): 125–138.

18. Odhiambo JA, Williams HC, Clayton TO, *et al.* (2009) Global variations in prevalence of eczema symptoms in children from ISAAC Phase Three. *J Allergy Clin Immunol* **124**(6): 1251–1258.e23.

19. Williams H, Stewart A, Von Mutius E, *et al.* (2008) Is eczema really on the increase worldwide? *J Allergy Clin Immunol* **121**(4): 947–954.e15.

20. Asher MI, Montefort S, Bjorksten B, *et al.* (2006) Worldwide time trends in the prevalence of symptoms of asthma, allergic rhinoconjunctivitis, and eczema in childhood: ISAAC Phases One and Three repeat multi-country cross-sectional surveys. *Lancet* **368**(9537): 733–743.

21. Guo Y, Li P, Tang J, *et al.* (2016) Prevalence of atopic dermatitis in Chinese children aged 1–7 years *Sci Rep* **6**: 29751.

22. Wang X, Li LF, Zhao DY, *et al.* (2016) Prevalence and clinical features of atopic dermatitis in China. *Biomed Res Int* **2016**: 2568301.

23. Wang X, Shi XD, Li LF, *et al.* (2017) Prevalence and clinical features of adult atopic dermatitis in tertiary hospitals of China. *Medicine (Baltimore)* **96**(11): e6317.

24. Shaw TE, Currie GP, Koudelka CW, *et al.* (2011) Eczema prevalence in the United States: Data from the 2003 National Survey of Children's Health. *J Invest Dermatol* **131**(1): 67–73.

25. Murray CJL, Vos T, Lozano R, *et al.* (2012) Disability-adjusted life years (DALYs) for 291 diseases and injuries in 21 regions, 1990–2010: A systematic analysis for the Global Burden of Disease Study 2010. *Lancet* **380**(9859): 2197–2223.

26. Simpson EL, Bieber T, Eckert L, *et al.* (2016) Patient burden of moderate to severe atopic dermatitis (AD): Insights from a phase 2b clinical trial of dupilumab in adults. *J Am Acad Dermatol* **74**(3): 491–498.

27. Drucker AM, Wang AR, Li WQ, *et al.* (2017) The burden of atopic dermatitis: Summary of a report for the National Eczema Association. *J Invest Dermatol* **137**(1): 26–30.
28. Chamlin SL, Frieden IJ, Williams ML, *et al.* (2004) Effects of atopic dermatitis on young American children and their families. *Pediatrics* **114**(3): 607–611.
29. Whiteley J, Emir B, Seitzman R, *et al.* (2016) The burden of atopic dermatitis in US adults: Results from the 2013 National Health and Wellness Survey. *Curr Med Res Opin* **32**(10): 1645–1651.
30. Chernyshov PV. (2016) Stigmatization and self-perception in children with atopic dermatitis. *Clin Cosmet Investig Dermatol* **9**: 159–166.
31. Lawson V, Lewis-Jones MS, Finlay AY, *et al.* (1998) The family impact of childhood atopic dermatitis: The Dermatitis Family Impact Questionnaire. *Br J Dermatol* **138**(1): 107–113.
32. Mancini AJ, Kaulback K, Chamlin SL. (2008) The socioeconomic impact of atopic dermatitis in the United States: A systematic review. *Pediatr Dermatol* **25**(1): 1–6.
33. Eckert L, Gupta S, Amand C, *et al.* (2018) The burden of atopic dermatitis in US adults: Health care resource utilization data from the 2013 National Health and Wellness Survey. *J Am Acad Dermatol* **78**(1): 54–61.e1.
34. Silverberg JI. (2015) Health care utilization, patient costs, and access to care in US adults with eczema: A population-based study. *JAMA Dermatol* **151**(7): 743–752.
35. Narla S, Hsu DY, Thyssen JP, *et al.* (2017) Inpatient financial burden of atopic dermatitis in the United States. *J Invest Dermatol* **137**(7): 1461–1467.
36. Jenner N, Campbell J, Marks R. (2004) Morbidity and cost of atopic eczema in Australia. *Aust J Dermatol* **45**(1): 16–22.
37. Zuberbier T, Orlow SJ, Paller AS, *et al.* (2006) Patient perspectives on the management of atopic dermatitis. *J Allergy Clin Immunol* **118**(1): 226–232.
38. Flohr C, Mann J. (2014) New insights into the epidemiology of childhood atopic dermatitis. *Allergy* **69**(1): 3–16.
39. Kantor R, Silverberg JI. (2017) Environmental risk factors and their role in the management of atopic dermatitis. *Expert Rev Clin Immunol* **13**(1): 15–26.
40. Mao W, Mao J, Zhang J, *et al.* (2014) Atopic eczema: A disease modulated by gene and environment. *Front Biosci (Landmark Ed)* **19**: 707–717.

41. Nutten S. (2015) Atopic dermatitis: Global epidemiology and risk factors. *Ann Nutr Metab*: 8–16.
42. Garg N, Silverberg JI. (2015) Epidemiology of childhood atopic dermatitis. *Clin Dermatol* **33**(3): 281–288.
43. D'Auria E, Banderali G, Barberi S, *et al.* (2016) Atopic dermatitis: Recent insight on pathogenesis and novel therapeutic target. *Asian Pac J Allergy Immunol* **34**(2): 98–108.
44. Bisgaard H, Simpson A, Palmer CN, *et al.* (2008) Gene-environment interaction in the onset of eczema in infancy: Filaggrin loss-of-function mutations enhanced by neonatal cat exposure. *PLoS Med* **5**(6): e131.
45. Lee JY, Seo JH, Kwon JW, *et al.* (2012) Exposure to gene-environment interactions before 1 year of age may favor the development of atopic dermatitis. *Int Arch Allergy Immunol* **157**(4): 363–371.
46. Kahr N, Naeser V, Stensballe LG, *et al.* (2015) Gene-environment interaction in atopic diseases: A population-based twin study of early-life exposures. *Clin Respir J* **9**(1): 79–86.
47. Sullivan M, Silverberg NB. (2017) Current and emerging concepts in atopic dermatitis pathogenesis. *Clin Dermatol* **35**(4): 349–353.
48. Fiset PO, Leung DY, Hamid Q. (2006) Immunopathology of atopic dermatitis. *J Allergy Clin Immunol* **118**(1): 287–290.
49. Eyerich K, Novak N. (2013) Immunology of atopic eczema: Overcoming the Th1/Th2 paradigm. *Allergy* **68**(8): 974–982.
50. Agrawal R, Wisniewski JA, Woodfolk JA. (2011) The role of regulatory T cells in atopic dermatitis. *Curr Probl Dermatol* **41**: 112–124.
51. Roesner LM, Floess S, Witte T, *et al.* (2015) Foxp3(+) regulatory T cells are expanded in severe atopic dermatitis patients. *Allergy* **70**(12): 1656–1660.
52. Hinz D, Bauer M, Roder S, *et al.* (2012) Cord blood Tregs with stable FOXP3 expression are influenced by prenatal environment and associated with atopic dermatitis at the age of one year. *Allergy* **67**(3): 380–389.
53. Reefer AJ, Satinover SM, Solga MD, *et al.* (2008) Analysis of CD25hiCD4+ "regulatory" T-cell subtypes in atopic dermatitis reveals a novel T(H)2-like population. *J Allergy Clin Immunol* **121**(2): 415–422.e3.
54. Eichenfield LF, Ellis CN, Mancini AJ, *et al.* (2012) Atopic dermatitis: Epidemiology and pathogenesis update. *Semin Cutan Med Surg* **31**(Suppl 3): S3–S5.
55. Janssens M, Van Smeden J, Gooris GS, *et al.* (2012) Increase in short-chain ceramides correlates with an altered lipid organization and decreased barrier function in atopic eczema patients. *J Lipid Res* **53**(12): 2755–2766.

56. Schlievert PM, Strandberg KL, Lin YC, *et al.* (2010) Secreted virulence factor comparison between methicillin-resistant and methicillin-sensitive *Staphylococcus aureus*, and its relevance to atopic dermatitis. *J Allergy Clin Immunol* **125**(1): 39–49.

57. Ong PY. (2014) New insights in the pathogenesis of atopic dermatitis. *Pediatr Res* **75**(1–2): 171–175.

58. Cardona ID, Cho SH, Leung DY. (2006) Role of bacterial superantigens in atopic dermatitis: Implications for future therapeutic strategies. *Am J Clin Dermatol* **7**(5): 273–279.

59. Wang L, Li LF. (2016) Clinical application of the UK Working Party's Criteria for the Diagnosis of Atopic Dermatitis in the Chinese population by age group. *Chin Med J (Engl)* **129**(23): 2829–2833.

60. Hanifin J, Rajka G. (1980) Diagnostic features of atopic dermatitis. *Acta Dermato-venereologica* **60**(Suppl 92): 44–47.

61. Williams H, Burney P, Hay R, *et al.* (1994) The UK Working Party's diagnostic criteria for atopic dermatitis. I. Derivation of a minimum set of discriminators for atopic dermatitis. *Br J Dermatol* **131**: 383–396.

62. Williams H, Burney P, Pembroke A, *et al.* (1994) The UK Working Party's diagnostic criteria for atopic dermatitis. III. Independent hospital validation. *Br J Dermatol* **131**: 406–416.

63. Kim JE, Kim HJ, Lew BL, *et al.* (2015) Consensus guidelines for the treatment of atopic dermatitis in Korea (Part I): General management and topical treatment. *Ann Dermatol* **27**(5): 563–577.

64. Eichenfield LF, Tom WL, Berger TG, *et al.* (2014) Guidelines of care for the management of atopic dermatitis: Section 2. Management and treatment of atopic dermatitis with topical therapies. *J Am Acad Dermatol* **71**(1): 116–132.

65. Sidbury R, Davis DM, Cohen DE, *et al.* (2014) Guidelines of care for the management of atopic dermatitis: Section 3. Management and treatment with phototherapy and systemic agents. *J Am Acad Dermatol* **71**(2): 327–349.

66. Sidbury R, Tom WL, Bergman JN, *et al.* (2014) Guidelines of care for the management of atopic dermatitis: Section 4. Prevention of disease flares and use of adjunctive therapies and approaches. *J Am Acad Dermatol* **71**(6): 1218–1233.

67. Wollenberg A, Oranje A, Deleuran M, *et al.* (2016) ETFAD/EADV Eczema task force 2015 position paper on diagnosis and treatment of atopic dermatitis in adult and paediatric patients. *J Eur Acad Dermatol Venereol* **30**(5): 729–747.

68. Saeki H, Nakahara T, Tanaka A, *et al.* (2016) Clinical practice guidelines for the management of atopic dermatitis 2016. *J Dermatol* **43**(10): 1117–1145.

69. 中华医学会皮肤性病学分会免疫学组, 特应性皮炎协作研究中心. (2014) 中国特应性皮炎诊疗指南 （2014版）. 中华皮肤科杂志 **47**(7): 511–514.

70. Kim JE, Kim HJ, Lew BL, *et al.* (2015) Consensus guidelines for the treatment of atopic dermatitis in Korea (Part II): Systemic treatment. *Ann Dermatol* **27**(5): 578–592.

71. Rubel D, Thirumoorthy T, Soebaryo RW, *et al.* (2013) Consensus guidelines for the management of atopic dermatitis: An Asia-Pacific perspective. *J Dermatol* **40**(3): 160–171.

72. Reljic V, Gazibara T, Nikolic M, *et al.* (2017) Parental knowledge, attitude, and behavior toward children with atopic dermatitis. *Int J Dermatol* **56**(3): 314–323.

73. Mohan GC, Lio PA. (2015) Comparison of dermatology and allergy guidelines for atopic dermatitis management. *JAMA Dermatol* **151**(9): 1009–1013.

74. The Royal Children's Hospital Melbourne. Skin infections: Bleach baths. Available from: https://www.rch.org.au/kidsinfo/fact_sheets/Skin_infections_-_bleach_baths/.

75. Ellis CN, Mancini AJ, Paller AS, *et al.* (2012) Understanding and managing atopic dermatitis in adult patients. *Semin Cutan Med Surg* **31**(Suppl 3): S18–S22.

2

Atopic Dermatitis in Chinese Medicine

OVERVIEW

Chinese medicine therapy can benefit atopic dermatitis by controlling the disease and reducing, or delaying, the risk of recurrence. This chapter will discuss the terminology, aetiology and pathogenesis, syndrome differentiation and treatments including Chinese herbal medicine, acupuncture and *tuina* 推拿 in current Chinese medicine textbooks and guidelines.

Introduction

Atopic dermatitis is known by several Chinese terms. The term *si wan feng* 四弯风 is one of the most well-known terms, as it describes the location where atopic dermatitis most commonly occurs in adults and adolescents. *Si wan feng* 四弯风 is the official term in the *Guidelines for Chinese Medicine Diagnosis and Treatment* 中医病证诊断疗效标准, published in 1994 by the State Administration of Traditional Chinese Medicine.[1] The term can be translated as 'four bends wind' or 'wind of four fossae', referring to the rash appearance on flexural surfaces. Other common terms for atopic dermatitis include *te ying xing pi yan* 特应性皮炎, *nai xuan* 奶癣 and *tai lian chuang* 胎敛疮.

Aetiology and Pathogenesis

Early references to the aetiology of atopic dermatitis can be found in *Wai Ke Zheng Zong* 外科正宗 (c. 1617). *Nai xuan* 奶癣 occurred when 'parents eat spicy food during pregnancy and deliver the heat to the baby; this flares all over the body after birth.' This passage shows the early understanding that infantile atopic dermatitis can be caused by improper diet during pregnancy, where heat can be transferred from the mother to the baby *in utero*. This is the origin of the Chinese medicine (CM) syndrome of foetal toxicity/heat.

In the Qing dynasty book *Wai Ke Xin Fa Yao Jue* 外科心法要诀 (c. 1742), *si wan feng* 四弯风 was said to linger and occur monthly, and was caused by evil wind. A later book from the Qing dynasty, *Yang Ke Jie Jing* 疡科捷径 (c. 1831), describes *si wan feng* 四弯风 as occurring 'at the popliteal fossa every year, is itchy and spreads like ringworm. The exterior is affected by wind evil with damp-heat....' These passages suggest that in the Qing dynasty, external wind pathogen and internal damp-heat were understood to underlie the aetiology for atopic dermatitis.

While differences exist in contemporary literature in relation to the aetiology and pathogenesis for atopic dermatitis, there is agreement on two important aspects: (1) congenital deficiency and (2) Spleen deficiency, and consequently failure of the transforming and transporting functions of the Spleen. In relation to congenital deficiency, the uterine environment is considered to be affected by the diet and emotions of the mother during pregnancy. Excessive intake of fatty and greasy food, excess of the five emotions or depression during pregnancy can lead to heat that is transferred to the foetus. This results in innate deficiency and excessive heat constitution in the unborn child.

A variety of factors can cause Spleen deficiency and dysfunction. Therefore, the treatments of atopic dermatitis normally focus on strengthening the Spleen. Improper feeding or malnutrition after birth can lead to failure of the Spleen in transforming and transporting food and fluids. The Spleen is responsible for generating *qi* and Blood, that is, postnatal essence. If the Spleen fails to function properly, the skin will not be nourished with sufficient *qi* and Blood, and thickening and dryness of the skin will occur.

Dampness is one of the most important factors in the occurrence of atopic dermatitis. Dampness is usually related to Spleen deficiency and the Spleen's failure to transform fluids. When the

Spleen fails to transform and transport, fluids and dampness will accumulate in the skin and atopic dermatitis will occur. As described in *Su Wen — Zhi Zhen Yao Da Lun* 素问·至真要大论 (Tang dynasty), 'all dampness swellings are caused by Spleen dysfunction.' Dampness will originate in the interior and smoulder in the body and skin.[2] Dampness is sticky and stagnant in nature, and syndromes of dampness are normally complex and difficult to recover from, which explains why atopic dermatitis has a long time course with frequent relapses.

In addition, hyperactive Heart *qi* in infants, or exuberant Heart fire from the external environment can transfer from the Heart to the Spleen (transfer of illness from 'mother' to 'son' in the five elements). Both the Heart and Spleen can be attacked at the same time.[3] When dampness collects in the Spleen for a long time and consumes fluids and Blood, Blood deficiency will generate wind and dryness and the skin will not be nourished. Furthermore, when externally contracted wind, dampness or heat combine with internal deficiency, this can lead to atopic dermatitis as well. Spleen deficiency plays a very important role throughout the development of atopic dermatitis.[2]

Syndrome Differentiation and Treatments

Atopic dermatitis diagnosis and treatment were not standardised until the publication of *Guidelines for Chinese Medicine Diagnosis and Treatment* 中医病证诊断疗效标准 by the State Administration of Traditional Chinese Medicine in 1994.[1] In *Guidelines*, the official CM name was defined as *si wan feng* 四弯风, with two syndrome differentiation types: wind-dampness collects in the skin and Blood deficiency with wind-dryness. The significance of the Spleen in atopic dermatitis was highlighted in later guidelines, including the 2011 *Atopic Dermatitis Clinical Practice Guidelines* 特应性皮炎中医临床实践指南 by the China Academy of China Medical Sciences[2] and the 2013 *Expert's Consensus on Chinese Medicine Diagnosis and Treatment for Atopic Dermatitis* 特应性皮炎中医诊疗方案专家共识 by the Association for Dermatology of the China Association of

Traditional Chinese Medicine.[3] Further research showed the interplay of these syndromes. In a review of theoretical and clinical literature related to atopic dermatitis syndrome differentiation from 1979 to 2012, the main syndrome was found to be Spleen deficiency combined with dampness or Blood dryness.[4]

The following guidelines and tertiary textbooks were referenced in this chapter: *Evidence-based Clinical Practice Guidelines* 特应性皮炎中医临床实践指南 (2011),[2] *Experts' Advice on Chinese Medicine Diagnosis and Treatment for Atopic Dermatitis* 特应性皮炎中医诊疗方案专家共识 (2013),[3] *Clinical Application Guide for Chinese Patent Drugs—Dermatology* 中成药临床应用指南•皮肤病分册 (2017),[5] *Chinese Medicine Surgery* 中医外科学 (1986, 2001, 2002, 2015, 2016),[6–10] and *Surgery of Integrated Traditional and Western Medicine* 中西医结合皮肤性病学 (2012, 2017).[11,12]

Textbooks and guidelines recommend oral Chinese herbal medicine (CHM) treatment based on the five key syndromes of atopic dermatitis. Topical CHM treatments are prescribed according to the appearance of the rash. A summary of CM syndromes and treatments can be found in Table 2.1.

Table 2.1. Summary of Oral Chinese Herbal Medicines for Atopic Dermatitis

Syndrome Differentiation	Treatment Principle	Formula
Heat accumulation in the Heart and Spleen	Clear the Heart and guide out heat.	Modified *San xin dao chi yin* 三心导赤饮[3,6,11,12]
Spleen deficiency with Heart heat	Clear the Heart and nourish the Spleen.	Modified *Pei tu qing xin fang* 培土清心方[3,6,11,12]
Spleen deficiency with dampness retention	Strengthen the Spleen and resolve dampness.	Modified *Xiao er hua shi tang* 小儿化湿汤加减[3,6,11,12]
Wind-dampness encumbering the skin	Dispel wind and damp.	Modified *Xiao feng san* 消风散加减[2]
Blood deficiency with wind-dryness	Nourish Blood and dispel wind.	Modified *Dang gui yin zi* 当归饮子加减[3,6,11,12]

Note: The use of some herbs may be restricted in some countries. In addition, some herbs are restricted under the provisions of the Convention on International Trade in Endangered Species of Wild Fauna and Flora (CITES). Readers are advised to comply with relevant regulations.

Oral Chinese Herbal Medicine Treatment Based on Syndrome Differentiation

Heat Accumulation in the Heart and Spleen 心脾积热证

Clinical manifestations: Facial erythema, papules and scaling skin with yellow crusts on the face or scalp. Exudate may be present. The rash may spread to the trunk and limbs, and children may be unsettled. Other symptoms may include hard/dry stool and dark urine. The skin on the forefinger appears purple to the *qi guan* 气关 area, and the pulse is rapid. This syndrome is common in children in the acute phase of atopic dermatitis.

Treatment principle: Clear the Heart and guide out heat 清心导赤.

Formula: Modified *San xin dao chi yin* 三心导赤饮.[3,6,11,12]

Herbs: *Lian qiao xin* 连翘心, *zhi zi xin* 栀子心, *lian zi xin* 莲子心, *xuan shen* 玄参, *sheng di huang* 生地黄, *che qian zi* 车前子, *chan tui* 蝉蜕, *deng xin cao* 灯心草, *fu ling* 茯苓 and *gan cao* 甘草.

Main actions of herbs: *Lian qiao xin, zhi zi xin, lian zi xin, deng xin cao* clear Heart and eliminate irritability; *che qian zi* clears heat and facilitates the water pathways with *deng xin cao; deng xin cao* promotes urination. *Sheng di huang* and *xuan shen* clear heat and cool the Blood, as well as nourish *yin* and generate fluid. *Fu ling* calms the spirit, strengthens the Spleen and leaches out dampness. *Chan tui* disperses all herbs to the skin, and *gan cao* clears heat, resolves toxicity and regulates all herbs.

Spleen Deficiency with Heart Heat 心火脾虚证

Clinical manifestations: Repeated episodes of erythema, swelling, blisters and cracked skin, with or without fluid exudate. Symptoms may appear on the face, neck, trunk, or in the cubital or popliteal fossa. Other symptoms include irritability and unsettled behaviour, poor sleep quality and decreased appetite. The tip of the tongue is red and the pulse is rapid. This syndrome is common in children in the acute phase.

Treatment principle: Clear the Heart and reinforce the Spleen 清心培土.

Formula: Modified *Pei tu qing xin fang* 培土清心方.[3,6,11,12]

Herbs: *Bai zhu* 白术, *shan yao* 山药, *yi yi ren* 薏苡仁, *lian qiao* 连翘, *deng xin cao* 灯心草, *dan zhu ye* 淡竹叶, *sheng di* 生地, *gou teng* 钩藤, *mu li* (decocted) 牡蛎 (先煎), *fang feng* 防风 and *gan cao* 甘草.

Main actions of herbs: *Bai zhu*, *yi yi ren* and *shan yao* strengthen the Spleen and draw out dampness. *Lian qiao*, *deng xin cao* and *sheng di* clear the Heart, nourish *yin qi* and calm irritability. *Dan zhu ye* guides out dampness-heat from urine, and *gou teng* calms the Liver and extinguishes wind to relieve itching. *Mu li* anchors the errant *yang*, nourishes *yin qi* and quiets the spirit; *gan cao* strengthens the Spleen, harmonises the middle burner and regulates all herbs.

Manufactured medicines: *Xiao er qi xing cha ke li* 小儿七星茶颗粒[5] promotes appetite, guides out stagnation, clears heat and settles anxiety.

Spleen Deficiency with Dampness Retention 脾虚湿蕴证

Clinical manifestations: Scattered papules, blisters and water blisters on limbs or other parts of the body. Other symptoms include fatigue and muscle weakness, decreased appetite and loose stools. The tongue body is pale with a white glossy coating, and the pulse is slow with pale colour on the forefinger. This syndrome is common in infants and children in the remission stage.

Treatment principle: Strengthen the Spleen and resolve dampness 健脾渗湿.

Formula: Modified *Xiao er hua shi tang* 小儿化湿汤加减.[3,6,11,12]

Herbs: *Cang zhu* 苍术, *fu ling* 茯苓, *chao mai ya* 炒麦芽, *chen pi* 陈皮, *ze xie* 泽泻, *hua shi* 滑石, *gan cao* 甘草, *chao bai zhu* 炒白术 and *chao yi yi ren* 炒薏苡仁.

Main actions of herbs: *Cang zhu*, *fu ling*, *chao mai ya*, *chen pi*, *chao bai zhu* and *chao yi yi ren* improve the Spleen's transporting function, while *ze xie*, *liu yi san* (*hua shi* and *gan cao*) draw out and resolve dampness.

Manufactured medicines: *Shen ling bai zhu san (wan)* 参苓白术散 (丸)[5] strengthens the Spleen and augments the *qi*. *Qi pi wan* 启脾丸[5] strengthens the Spleen and harmonises the Stomach.

Wind-dampness Encumbering the Skin 风湿蕴肤证

Clinical manifestations: Rash which can appear anywhere on the body, especially on the face and limbs. The rash appears as sparse or dense clusters of papules, and patches of skin become dry, flaky and itchy which are worse in windy weather. Other symptoms include dry mouth, itchy throat, red eyes and constipation. The tongue is red with little or dry coating, and the pulse is rapid, floating and slippery.

Treatment principle: Dispel wind and damp 祛风祛湿.

Formula: Modified *Xiao feng san* 消风散加减.[2]

Herbs: *Jing jie* 荆芥, *ku shen* 苦参, *zhi mu* 知母, *cang zhu* 苍术, *qiang huo* 羌活, *chan tui* 蝉蜕, *fang feng* 防风, *niu bang zi* 牛蒡子, *sheng di huang* 生地黄, *hu ma ren* 胡麻仁, *fu ling* 茯苓, *sheng shi gao* 生石膏 and *dang gui* 当归.

Main actions of herbs: *Jing jie, ku shen, niu bang zi* and *chan tui* disperse wind and clear pathogens from the exterior. *Cang zhu* dispels wind and dries dampness, and *ku shen* clears heat and dries dampness. *Sheng shi gao* and *zhi mu* clear heat and drain fire. *Dang gui, sheng di huang* and *hu ma ren* nourish and invigorate the Blood. *Gan cao* clears heat and toxicity, harmonises the middle burner and regulates all herbs.

Manufactured medicines: *Fang feng tong sheng wan* 防风通圣丸[2] releases the exterior and promotes the interior, and clears heat and toxicity.

Blood Deficiency with Wind-Dryness 血虚风燥证

Clinical manifestations: Very dry skin, and the affected patch of skin inside the elbows and knees becomes thick and leathery. The skin on the arms and legs becomes extremely itchy, and multiple excoriated lesions are caused by scratching. Other symptoms include pale face, normally slim build, poor sleep quality and dry stool. The tongue is pale, and the pulse is wiry and thready. This syndrome is common in adolescents and adults in the remission stage.

Treatment principle: Nourish Blood and dispel wind 养血祛风.

Formula: Modified *Dang gui yin zi* 当归饮子加减. [3,6,11,12]

Herbs: *Huang qi* 黄芪, *sheng di* 生地, *shu di* 熟地, *bai shao* 白芍, *dang gui* 当归, *chuan xiong* 川芎, *he shou wu* 何首乌, *bai ji li* 白蒺藜, *jing jie* 荆芥 and *fang fang* 防风.

Main actions of herbs: *Shu di, bai shao, dang gui, chuan xiong* and *he shou wu* enrich the *yin*, promote Blood and moisten the dryness. *Sheng di* clears heat and cools Blood; *jing jie, fang fang* and *bai ji li* dispel wind and relieve itching.

Manufactured medicines: *Run zao zhi yang* capsule 润燥止痒胶囊[5] nourishes Blood and enriches the *yin*, dispels wind and relieves itching, lubricates the intestines and unblocks the bowels. *Shi du qing* capsule 湿毒清胶囊[5] promotes Blood and moistens dryness, dispels wind and relieves itching.

Topical Chinese Herbal Medicine Treatment

Topical CHM can provide additional relief for atopic dermatitis. Topical treatments can be in various forms, such as lotions, creams and ointments. Treatments are selected based on the appearance of the rash, as described below.

Rashes, Papules or Blisters, without Exudate

A wash can be prepared by boiling 15 grams of *huang jing* 黄精 and 15 grams of *jin yin hua* 金银花 in two litres of water until the volume is reduced to 1.5 litres. Allow the liquid to cool, and wash the affected skin.[3,6,11,12] Manufactured treatments include *Chuan bai zhi yang* lotion 川百止痒洗剂 and *Chi shi zhi yang* ointment 除湿止痒软膏.[5]

Inflamed, Swollen and Cracked Skin with Exudate

When the rash is inflamed with exudate, increase the amount of *jin yin hua* 金银花 to 30 grams and add 15 grams of *gan cao* 甘草 to 15 grams of *huang jing* 黄精. Boil the herbs in two litres of water until the volume reduces to 1.5 litres. Once cool, the liquid can be used to wash the affected skin or as a cool compress. If symptoms worsen, a cool compress can be made by boiling *huang bai* 黄柏, *di yu* 地榆, *ma chi xian* 马齿苋 and *ye ju hua* 野菊花. This mixture will clear heat and toxicity, and alleviate the symptoms.[3,6,11,12] Between applications of cool compress, oil mixtures can be applied to the affected skin. Two mixtures are recommended in guidelines: (1) 5~10% *gan cao* oil 甘草油, *zi cao* oil 紫草油, or *qing dai* oil 青黛油,[3,6,11,12] and (2) *huang lian* oil 黄连油 and *zhe dan huang* oil 蛋黄油.[7-10] Manufactured products include *Fu fang huang bai* lotion 复方黄柏液 and *Pi fu kang* lotion 皮肤康洗液.[5,8]

Dry, Flaked, Thick and Leathery Skin

Applying moisturiser is an essential requirement for self-care of atopic dermatitis. Moisturiser should be applied at least twice daily. Herbal moisturisers include 5~10% *huang lian* ointment 黄连软膏, *Fu fang she zhi* ointment 复方蛇脂软膏 or other moisturizing ointments;[3,6,11,12] or *huang bai* cream 黄柏霜.[7-10] Manufactured products include *Qing peng* cream 青鹏乳膏 and *Hei dou liu you* ointment 黑豆馏油软膏.[5]

Acupuncture and Other Chinese Medicine Therapies

Acupuncture and auricular acupuncture can effectively control the symptoms of atopic dermatitis and relieve itching. *Tuina* 推拿 is particularly beneficial for patients under 12 years of age, but is not suitable for inflamed skin. Acupuncture, moxibustion, plum blossom needle therapy and *tuina* 推拿 have been recommended as treatments for atopic dermatitis.

Several important acupuncture points have been recommended for use with multiple intervention types. Actions of key acupuncture points are as follows[13]:

- LI11 *Quchi* 曲池: Clears heat, cools the Blood, eliminates wind, drains damp, alleviates itching and regulates *qi* and Blood.
- ST36 *Zusanli* 足三里: Harmonises the Stomach, strengthens the Spleen, resolves dampness, tonifies *qi*, nourishes Blood and *yin*, clears fire and calms the spirit.
- SP10 *Xuehai* 血海: Invigorates Blood, dispels stasis, cools Blood and benefits the skin.
- SP6 *Sanyinjiao* 三阴交: Tonifies the Stomach and Spleen, resolves dampness, invigorates Blood and calms the spirit.
- SP9 *Yinlingquan* 阴陵泉: Regulates the Spleen and resolves dampness.
- LI4 *Hegu* 合谷: Regulates *wei qi* 衛氣, expels wind and releases the exterior.
- LI15 *Jianyu* 肩髃: Dispels wind-damp, eliminates wind, regulates *qi* and Blood, and dissipates phlegm nodules.
- GV14 *Dazhui* 大椎: Expels wind and firms the exterior, clears heat, tonifies deficiency and pacifies wind.

A summary of interventions and acupuncture points can be found in Table 2.2.

Acupuncture

Four approaches have been described to select acupuncture points.[2] These include selecting points according to the affected meridian, syndrome differentiation and stage (acute or chronic), and selecting *Ashi* points 阿是穴. Electroacupuncture is recommended for *Ashi* points 阿是穴 and has been summarised in the 'Electroacupuncture' section below.

When selecting points according to the affected meridian, the main acupuncture points recommended in clinical guidelines are LI11 *Quchi* 曲池, BL40 *Weizhong* 委中 and SP10 *Xuehai* 血海.[2] Supplementary points can be selected from PC7 *Daling* 大陵, LI15

Table 2.2. Summary of Acupuncture Therapies and Other Chinese Medicine Therapies for Atopic Dermatitis

Intervention	Acupuncture Points; Body Area
Acupuncture[2,11]	**1. According to meridian** Main points: LI11 *Quchi* 曲池, BL40 *Weizhong* 委中 and SP10 *Xuehai* 血海. Supplementary points: PC7 *Daling* 大陵, LI15 *Jianyu* 肩髃 and PC3 *Quze* 曲泽. **2. According to syndrome** Main points: LI11 *Quchi* 曲池, ST36 *Zusanli* 足三里, SP6 *Sanyinjiao* 三阴交 and SP9 *Yinlingquan* 阴陵泉. Excess dampness: BL20 *Pishu* 脾俞, ST28 *Shuidao* 水道 and BL13 *Feishu* 肺俞. Spleen deficiency with dampness encumbrance: SP3 *Taibai* 太白, BL20 *Pishu* 脾俞 and BL21 *Weishu* 胃俞. Blood deficiency with wind-dryness: BL17 *Geshu* 膈俞, BL18 *Ganshu* 肝俞 and SP10 *Xuehai* 血海. **3. According to stage** Acute stage: GV14 *Dazhui* 大椎, LI11 *Quchi* 曲池, BL13 *Feishu* 肺俞, BL40 *Weizhong* 委中, SP10 *Xuehai* 血海, ST36 *Zusanli* 足三里, SP6 *Sanyinjiao* 三阴交 and SP9 *Yinlingquan* 阴陵泉. Chronic stage: SP10 *Xuehai* 血海, ST36 *Zusanli* 足三里, SP6 *Sanyinjiao* 三阴交 and SP9 *Yinlingquan* 阴陵泉.
Moxibustion[2]	Main points: LI11 *Quchi* 曲池 and SP10 *Xuehai* 血海. Supplementary points: LI15 *Jianyu* 肩髃, GB30 *Huantiao* 环跳, LI4 *Hegu* 合谷, GV20 *Baihui* 百会, GV14 *Dazhui* 大椎 and *Ashixue* 阿是穴 (itching spot).
Ear acupuncture[2]	CO14 *Fei* (Lung) 肺, TG2p *Shenshangxian* (Adrenal gland) 肾上腺, CO18 *Neifenmi* (Endocrine) 内分泌, CO13 *Pi* (Spleen) 脾, TF4 *Shenmen* 神门; zone for affected area.
Electroacupuncture[2]	Ashi points 阿是穴.
Plum blossom needle therapy[2]	LI11 *Quchi* 曲池, LI4 *Hegu* 合谷, and ST36 *Zusanli* 足三里; sides of the spine, local area.
Tuina 推拿[3,11]	Clear *Tian he shui* 天河水*, CV12 *Zhongwan* 中脘; Bladder meridian.

*Clearing *Tian he shui* 天河水 is a technique where two fingers are placed on the centre of the anterior wrist crease and rubbed up the centre of the forearm along the Pericardium meridian to PC3 *Quze* 曲泽 at the cubital crease. This process is repeated, always drawing the fingers upwards. Although not described as an acupuncture point, the centre of the wrist crease is likely to be PC7 *Daling* 大陵.

Jianyu 肩髃 and PC3 *Quze* 曲泽. Proximal and distal points may include CV1 *Huiyin* 会阴, CV3 *Zhongji* 中极, SP6 *Sanyinjiao* 三阴交, LR5 *Ligou* 蠡沟 and LR1 *Dadun* 大敦.

When selecting points according to syndrome differentiation, local lesions and points on the foot *Taiyang* 太陽 meridians are the main acupuncture points[2] e.g. LI11 *Quchi* 曲池, ST36 *Zusanli* 足三里, SP6 *Sanyinjiao* 三阴交 and SP9 *Yinlingquan* 阴陵泉. For excessive dampness, add BL20 *Pishu* 脾俞, ST28 *Shuidao* 水道 and BL13 *Feishu* 肺俞. For Spleen deficiency with dampness encumbrance, add SP3 *Taibai* 太白, BL20 *Pishu* 脾俞 and BL21 *Weishu* 胃俞. For Blood deficiency and wind-dryness, add BL17 *Geshu* 膈俞, BL18 *Ganshu* 肝俞 and SP10 *Xuehai* 血海. For severe itching, add GB20 *Fengchi* 风池, GV20 *Baihui* 百会 and EX-HN1 *Sishencong* 四神聪.

During flares of atopic dermatitis, acupuncture points should include GV14 *Dazhui* 大椎, LI11 *Quchi* 曲池, BL13 *Feishu* 肺俞, BL40 *Weizhong* 委中, SP10 *Xuehai* 血海, ST36 *Zusanli* 足三里, SP6 *Sanyinjiao* 三阴交 and SP9 *Yinlingquan* 阴陵泉. In the chronic stage, ST36 *Zusanli* 足三里, SP9 *Yinlingquan* 阴陵泉, LI11 *Quchi* 曲池 and SP10 *Xuehai* 血海 should be used.[2] Reinforcing techniques should be used in cases of deficiency, and reducing methods used in cases of excess. Treatment should be administered daily in the acute stage, and on alternate days in the chronic stage.

Moxibustion

The main points for moxibustion are LI11 *Quchi* 曲池 and SP10 *Xuehai* 血海.[2] Supplementary points can be added, and may include LI15 *Jianyu* 肩髃, GB30 *Huantiao* 环跳, LI4 *Hegu* 合谷, GV20 *Baihui* 百会, GV14 *Dazhui* 大椎 and *Ashixue* 阿是穴 (itching spot). Mild moxibustion should be applied to each acupuncture point for five to 15 minutes daily.

Ear Acupuncture

Select three to four ear acupuncture points from CO14 *Fei* (Lung) 肺, TG2p *Shenshangxian* (Adrenal gland) 肾上腺, CO18 *Neifenmi*

(Endocrine) 内分泌, CO13 *Pi* (Spleen) 脾 and TF4 *Shenmen* 神门, zones for the affected area.[2] Needles should be retained for 30 minutes and treatment provided daily.

Electroacupuncture

Apply electroacupuncture to local *Ashi* points 阿是穴 around the rash area.[2] Needles should be inserted obliquely around the rash area. Attach electrodes, and gradually increase the current until tolerable for the patient. Treatment should be applied for 20 minutes, once every day or every second day.

Plum Blossom Needle Therapy

Plum blossom needle therapy can be applied to these acupuncture points: LI11 *Quchi* 曲池, LI4 *Hegu* 合谷 and ST36 *Zusanli* 足三里, to both sides of the spine and to the affected area.[2] Plum blossom needle therapy can be applied with moderate intensity to acupuncture points, and can be applied with stronger intensity bilaterally on the thoracic and lumbar regions.

Tuina 推拿

In the acute stage, *tuina* 推拿 (Chinese massage) can be used to clear *Tian he shui* 天河水 (see note for Table 2.2), and applied to CV12 *Zhongwan* 中脘 and along the Bladder channel on the back. During the chronic stage, *mo fu* 摩腹 (rubbing exercise) can be applied to the abdomen, chiropractic therapy can be used, and kneading and pressing techniques applied to ST36 *Zusanli* 足三里.[3,11]

Other Management Strategies

As described earlier, bathing and moisturising are important components of overall care. Bathing should be restricted to five minutes, and patients should be advised to avoid alkaline detergents. Moisturiser should be applied immediately after bathing to protect the skin barrier and control atopic dermatitis. Suitable moisturisers should be applied at least twice daily.[2,3,6,7,9]

Triggers associated with the living environment should be avoided, including dramatic changes in ambient temperature and identified food and drug triggers. Patients should avoid ingested and inhaled allergens, as well as contact allergens such as wool, rough and irritating textiles, and tobacco. Patients should be advised to trim their nails regularly to minimise scratches on the skin.[2,3,6,7,9]

Patients can participate in their own health care by making changes to their diet and lifestyle. Diet is particularly important, as atopic dermatitis is closely related to the Spleen and Stomach. Making healthy choices can help to strengthen the Spleen. Patients should be advised to avoid spicy and irritable food.[2,3,6] Other factors that can reduce the severity and/or impact of atopic dermatitis include avoiding staying up late or getting overtired, avoiding stress, participating in regular exercise, and ensuring adequate fluid intake and fibre for bowel health. Where symptoms affect mental health, patients should be encouraged to seek professional support.[2,3,6,7]

References

1. 国家中医药管理局. (1994) 中医病证诊断疗效标准. 南京: 南京大学出版社.

2. 世界卫生组织西太区中医临床实践指南项目组. (2011) 特应性皮炎中医临床实践指南. 北京: 中国中医药出版社, pp. 24–36.

3. 中华中医药学会皮肤科专业委员会. (2013) 特应性皮炎中医诊疗方案专家共识. 中国中西医结合皮肤性病学杂志 **12**(1): 60–61.

4. 张冰, 梁碧欣, 吴元胜, 等. (2014) 基于数据挖掘技术的特应性皮炎辨治规律分析. 中华中医药学刊 **32**(5): 1029–1032.

5. 杨志波. (2017) 中成药临床应用指南•皮肤病分册. 北京: 中国中医药出版社, pp. 108–115.

6. 刘胜, 陈达灿. (2015) 中医外科学 (国家卫生和计划生育委员会 "十二五" 规划教程). 北京: 人民卫生出版社.

7. 陈红风. (2016) 中医外科学 (全国中医药行业高等教育"十三五"规划教材). 北京: 中国中医药出版社, p. 173.

8. 顾伯康. (1986) 中医外科学 (高等医药院校教材). 上海: 上海科学技术出版社, p. 140.

9. 陆德铭. (2001) 中医外科学 (普通高等教育中医药类规划教材). 上海: 上海科学技术出版社, pp. 141–142.

10. 李曰庆. (2002) 中医外科学 (新世纪全国高等中医药院校规划教材). 北京: 中国中医药出版社, pp. 185–186.

11. 陈德宇.(2012)中西医结合皮肤性病学(全国中医药行业高等教育"十二五"规划教材). 北京: 中国中医药出版社, pp. 188–191.

12. 李斌, 陈达灿. (2017) 中西医结合皮肤性病学 (全国中医药行业高等教育"十三五"规划教材). 北京: 中国中医药出版社.

13. Deadman P, Al-Khafaji M, Baker K. (2000) *A Manual of Acupuncture.* Journal of Chinese Medicine Publications, East Sussex, England.

3

Classical Chinese Medicine Literature

OVERVIEW

Contemporary clinical practice of Chinese medicine continues to develop, often guided by valuable information contained in the classical literature. This chapter reviews the historical literature relating to management of atopic dermatitis. Eleven search terms were used to identify references in the classical literature that were possibly related to atopic dermatitis. More than 500 citations were identified, and the information related to treatment reviewed. Oral and topical Chinese herbal medicine were important treatment choices for atopic dermatitis, while other Chinese medicine therapies were used less frequently.

Introduction

Chinese medicine (CM) has a long history. The earliest written records which show evidence of professional practice date back to the Spring and Autumn (770–476 BC) and Warring states (474–221 BC) periods. In these passages concepts such as *yin* and *yang* are evident, and therapeutic methods included the use of mugwort (*ai* 艾) for moxibustion, herbal decoctions and acupuncture.[1] These methods have been described throughout CM classical texts as treatments for many conditions, including skin conditions.

Atopic dermatitis is one of the most common skin conditions described in contemporary and classical CM texts. Many of the treatments used in clinical practice today have their origins in classical literature, and previous research has examined the historical development of atopic dermatitis in CM.[2,3] Research by Huang *et al.* (2011)[2]

consulted 24 books of historical significance to dermatology. Seventy-one citations considered relevant to atopic dermatitis were found in a variety of books, including general medical and surgical books. The predominant descriptions of the aetiology for this condition related to wind, dampness and toxic heat. Symptoms were typical of the current understanding of atopic dermatitis, and included itch, pain, exudate and dry lesions. External application of Chinese herbal medicine (CHM) was common, and the most common formulas were *Jie du xiong huang san* 解毒雄黄散 and *Wen ge san* 文蛤散.

Research by Tan in 2014[3] used the digitalised collection of more than 1,000 classical CM texts: the *Zhong Hua Yi Dian* (ZHYD 中华医典, Encyclopedia of Traditional Chinese Medicine).[4] In this research, 738 citations were identified for atopic dermatitis with the vast majority of citations describing management with CHM. The most common symptoms were itch, exudation and chronicity/recurrence, which are typical presentations of atopic dermatitis. The most common formulas for topical application were *Run ji gao* 润肌膏, *San miao san* 三妙散 and *Wu yun gao* 乌云膏, and the most frequently used oral (systemic) formula was *Xiao feng dao chi tang* 消风导赤汤.

The key formulas for topical application in research by Huang *et al.*[2] differed from those found by Tan.[3] This is likely due to the research by Huang *et al.* being limited to 24 books. The collection of books in the ZHYD is the largest currently available, and is representative of other large collections of the classical and pre-modern CM literature.[5,6] The edition used by Tan[3] has since been updated, and the collection now includes in excess of 1,100 books. In order to review a sample of the classical and pre-modern literature, we conducted further searches using the ZHYD.

Search Terms

In contemporary texts, the terms *te ying xing pi yan* 特应性皮炎 and *si wan feng* 四弯风 are frequently used to describe atopic dermatitis.[7] In addition to these terms, other terms have been used throughout classical CM literature. Terms such as *nai xuan* 奶癣 and *tai lian chuang* 胎㿜疮 are synonymous with infantile eczema. Other terms such as *jin yin chuang* 浸淫疮 are more general in describing eczema-like conditions.

In order to identify citations in classical literature related to atopic dermatitis, a comprehensive list of terms was collated by searching dermatological and general medical textbooks and dictionaries. These included: *Zhong Yi Pi Fu Bing Zheng Zhuang Jian Bie Zhen Duan Yu Zhi Liao* 中医皮肤病症状鉴别诊断与治疗 (Differential Diagnosis of Symptoms and Treatment in Dermatology of Traditional Chinese Medicine, 2015),[8] Gu Bohua's *Zhong Yi Wai Ke Xue* 中医外科学 (Surgery of Traditional Chinese Medicine, 1987),[9] and Zhao Shanghua's *Zhong Yi Wai Ke Xue* 中医外科学 (Surgery of Traditional Chinese Medicine, 2002).[10] In addition, the selection of search terms drew on the research of Huang *et al.*,[2] who have conducted similar work previously.

Through this process, a list of 11 terms was produced. Test searches were conducted in the ZHYD to determine the accuracy of these terms in identifying potentially relevant citations, and to get an estimate of the number of citations to be considered for inclusion. The search terms and possible translations are described in Table 3.1. The term *te ying xing pi yan* 特应性皮炎 was not included as a search

Table 3.1.   Search Terms and Possible Meaning

Pinyin	Chinese Characters	Possible Translation/Meaning
Jin yin chuang	浸淫疮	General effused eczema
Lian mei chuang 1	恋眉疮	Infantile seborrheic eczema
Lian mei chuang 2	炼眉疮	Infantile seborrheic eczema
Lian yin chuang	炼银疮	Infantile seborrheic eczema
Nai xuan	奶癣	Milk tinea
Ru xian	乳癣	Infantile eczema
Si wan feng	四弯风	Four bends wind (wind of four fossae)
Su chuang	粟疮	Millet sore
Tai lian chuang	胎㿂疮	Infantile eczema
Tai xuan	胎癣	Infantile eczema
Xue feng chuang	血风疮	Blood-wind sores

term, as this is a modern term and was unlikely to identify citations in classical and pre-modern literature.

Some of the terms selected were used for atopic dermatitis in any age, while others were specific to infants, such as *nai xuan/tai xuan* 奶癣/胎癣. The term *nai xuan* 奶癣 can be literally translated as 'milk tinea' and may relate to infantile eczema.[3] Other terms were more descriptive of symptoms. For example, *su chuang* 粟疮 could be translated as 'millet sore,' suggesting lesions appeared as small grains, while *si wan feng* 四弯风 refers to lesions in the four fossa. Other terms were more closely related to aetiology, while *xue feng chuang* 血风疮 referred to a rash due to wind affecting the Blood.

Procedures for Search, Data Coding and Data Analysis

Each term was entered into the ZHYD search fields and the search results were downloaded to spreadsheets (Fig. 3.1). A 'citation' was defined as a distinct passage of text referring to one, or more, of the search terms. Codes were allocated for types of citations, books and the dynasties in which they were written according to the procedures described in May *et al.* (2013).[6] Books written after 1949 were excluded.

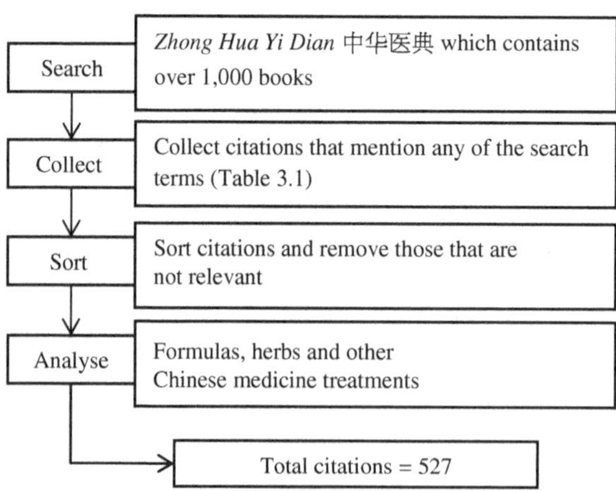

Fig. 3.1. Classical literature citations

The number of hits returned for each search term was recorded and summed to provide the total number of hits. Some citations were located by two or more of the selected search terms. In this instance, the additional terms which identified the duplicate citation were recorded and the duplicate citation was removed from the dataset. Further screening was conducted to remove irrelevant citations. Citations were excluded if they were not related to skin conditions or atopic dermatitis, were CM dictionary citations, were herb citations which were pharmacopeia-type entries, or were not relevant.

The remaining citations were reviewed to identify the best descriptions of the condition and its aetiology or pathogenesis; these were selected for presentation in this chapter. Information about CM syndrome differentiation was extracted. Citations were reviewed to determine the likelihood of them representing atopic dermatitis. Inclusion criteria were based on similar work conducted previously,[2] and related to four characteristic symptoms of atopic dermatitis:

- Itch.
- Skin rash or skin dryness.
- Rash location (elbow, knee, head, face, neck).
- Chronicity or relapse.

The presence or absence of each of these symptoms was recorded, and a judgment made as to the likelihood of them relating to atopic dermatitis. Citations which described any two or more of these four symptoms were considered as 'possible' references to atopic dermatitis. Citations which described any three or more for the four symptoms were considered 'most likely' to be atopic dermatitis. Citations which described only one of the four symptoms were considered to have insufficient information to make a judgment. Citations which contained no information or inadequate information to judge the likelihood of being atopic dermatitis were also excluded.

Citations were further reviewed to identify CM treatments, and those which did not describe treatment were excluded from further analysis. The final data set included citations considered to refer to atopic dermatitis, which described CM treatments

(CHM, acupuncture and related therapies, or other CM therapies). When a citation described multiple treatments, each treatment was considered as a separate citation for calculation of formulas, herbs or acupuncture points. Citations which were pharmacopeia-type entries were reviewed for eligibility. Pharmacopeia entries which mentioned the name of the condition but did not include a detailed description of the condition or information about treatment were excluded from further analysis. Pharmacopeia entries which included a description of the condition, with or without reference to other herbs, were included. Single acupuncture points were reviewed in a similar manner. Data are presented for the frequencies of identified formulas, herbs and acupuncture points for 'possible' and 'most likely' atopic dermatitis citations.

Search Results

Searches of both the headings and body of the text of the ZHYD resulted in 527 hits (Table 3.2). Two terms identified the majority of citations: *Jin yin chuang* 浸淫疮 (180 hits, 34.2%) and *xue feng chuang* 血风疮 (141 hits, 26.8%). Six terms identified ten or fewer

Table 3.2.   Hit Frequency by Search Term

Pinyin	Chinese Characters	Hit Frequency: *n* (%)
Jin yin chuang	浸淫疮	180 (34.2)
Xue feng chuang	血风疮	141 (26.8)
Su chuang	粟疮	80 (15.2)
Nai xuan	奶癣	44 (8.3)
Ru xuan	乳癣	30 (5.7)
Si wan feng	四弯风	10 (1.9)
Tai xuan	胎癣	10 (1.9)
Lian mei chuang 1	恋眉疮	10 (1.9)
Lian yin chuang	炼银疮	9 (1.7)
Lian mei chuang 2	炼眉疮	7 (1.3)
Tai lian chuang	胎瀲疮	6 (1.1)

citations, suggesting that these terms were not commonly used to describe atopic dermatitis-like conditions in classical books.

Citations which were not related to the condition, and those with insufficient information to make a judgment, were excluded from further analysis. Citations that were entries in CM dictionaries, or that were pharmacopeia-style herb entries without a description of atopic dermatitis, were excluded, as were citations from books published after 1949. After exclusion of duplicates, irrelevant citations and those with insufficient information to make a judgment, 110 citations were considered 'possibly' or 'most likely' to relate to atopic dermatitis. Twelve of these provided a description of atopic dermatitis but did not describe treatment. Fifty-four citations described two or more CM treatments, with many describing several. One citation from the Ming dynasty book *Yi Xue Ru Men* 医学入门 (c. 1575) described 11 different herbal treatments. When citations, including multiple treatments, were separated for analysis, the final number of treatment citations was 271. The vast majority related to CHM, and three citations related to other CM therapies.

Definitions of Atopic Dermatitis

Early CM texts contained rich descriptions of skin conditions likely to be atopic dermatitis. Several citations described symptoms in babies, and offered treatment options with CHM. In *Wai Ke Xin Fa Yao Jue* 外科心法要诀 (c. 1742) symptoms found on the top of the head or tip of the brow were described as white debris-like scabies accompanied by an itch (痒起白屑, 形如癣疥). These symptoms were further elaborated and differentiated in a passage by Zheng Yutan 鄭玉壇 in *Tong Yuan Yi Shu — Wai Ke* 彤园医书 (外科) (c. 1796). Zheng describes the rash as being dry at the outset, but when babies are washed in water that is too hot the rash is aggravated and papules, itch and exudation spread all over the body. This type was considered wet-type atopic dermatitis. Both types can be treated with the formula *Xiao feng dao chi tang* 俱服消风导赤汤 (初系干癣, 若误用热水烫洗, 致皮肤起粟, 瘙痒无度, 黄水浸淫, 延及遍身, 即成湿癣。俱服消风导赤汤), and a second formula (*Wu fu hua du dan* 五福化毒丹) can be added where the skin is burning, hot, red and flaking. This passage also describes different topical ointments for dry-type atopic dermatitis (use *Run ji gao* 润肌膏), wet-type atopic dermatitis (use *Er sheng gao* 二神膏) and wet-type with severe itching (use *Wu yun gao* 乌云膏).

An earlier citation from the Ming dynasty described *nai xuan* 奶癣 as appearing on the head, face and all over the body after birth [*Wai Ke Zheng Zong* 外科正宗, (c. 1617)]. Symptoms included thick fluid exudate, sleep disturbance and endless scratching due to itch. These symptoms could be treated with *Wen ge san* 文蛤散 or *Xiong huang jie du san* 解毒雄黄散, or *Cui yun san* 翠云散 when symptoms were serious. In children, skin lesions were described as long or round in shape, and grew gradually [*Pu Ji Fang* 普济方 Volumes 358–480, (c. 1406)]. Lesions could occur on the face and were rough and dry (皮如甲错干燥). Skin rash was accompanied by itch, yellow exudate after scratching, and a stuffy feeling when warm (暖则痒闷, 搔之即黄汁出, 又或在面上).

In other citations, the location of atopic dermatitis was more typical of that reported in children and adults. In a passage from *Yang Ke Jie Jing* 疡科捷径 (c. 1831), *si wan feng* 四弯风 occurred on the popliteal fossa each year and was characterised by intense itch and exudate that spread gradually to have the appearance of tinea. This case was considered as a combination of two syndromes — external wind and internal dampness-heat. Treatment with *Xiao feng san* 消风散 provided relief (四弯风, 岁腿弯生, 淫痒滋延似癣形。外受风邪兼湿热, 消风散妙最为灵).

Perhaps one of the most detailed descriptions of atopic dermatitis was found in *Wai Ke Xin Fa Yao Jue* 外科心法要诀 (c. 1742). This passage described symptoms and rash site, and provided a treatment option with CHM, together with an explanation of the treatment. *Si wan feng* 四弯风 occurred on both sides of the popliteal fossa and the ankles. The disease relapsed every month and was difficult to cure. The appearance was like wind-tinea, caused by wind invasion of the skin. Itch was excessive, scratching released fluids (exudation) and lesions were wet in appearance. Topical wash could be applied by boiling a soup with one litre of barley. External use of *San miao san* 三妙散 would remove damp, kill insects and relieve itching. (四弯风, 生腿脚弯, 每月一发最缠绵, 形如风癣风邪袭, 搔破成疮痒难堪。【注】此证生在两腿弯, 脚弯, 每月一发, 形如风癣, 属风邪袭入腠理而成。 其痒无度, 搔破津水, 形如湿癣. 法宜大麦一升熬汤, 先熏后洗; 次搽三妙散, 渗湿杀虫, 其痒即止, 缓缓取效.) This passage is often cited in contemporary CM texts due to its detailed description of the condition and treatment.

Descriptions of the Aetiology of Atopic Dermatitis

Recent scientific research has highlighted the importance of genetic factors, the intrauterine environment, and the first year of life in the development of atopic dermatitis (see Chapter 1).[11,12] The intrauterine environment has long been regarded as important for foetal growth and development in CM. In CM, Kidney *jing* 精 is inherited from the parents and the quality of their Kidney *jing* 精 at the time of conception is passed on to the child.[13] Some of the early descriptions of the 'most likely' cases of atopic dermatitis alluded to these understandings. A passage from *Wai Ke Zheng Zong* 外科正宗 (c. 1617) introduces foetal heat as a syndrome related to atopic dermatitis. The passage states that heat can be transferred from the parents to the foetus when the parents tend to eat strong-flavoured food (母食五辛, 父餐炙爆, 遗热与儿). This is seen as one of the causes of atopic dermatitis. Another section of the *Wai Ke Zheng Zong* 外科正宗 elaborates on this, stating that the heat affects the Blood of the foetus (Blood heat). Finally, wind invasion after birth is seen as another factor in the development of atopic dermatitis (由胎中血热, 落草受风缠绵).

The early care of the infant was also thought to contribute to the development of atopic dermatitis. Washing the baby with water that is too hot was said to result in eruption of skin papules and excessive itch, with yellow watery exudate that spreads all over the body (有误用烫洗, 皮肤起粟, 搔痒无度, 黄水浸淫, 延及遍身, 即成湿癣). Environmental exposure was also highlighted in a passage from Volumes 358–480 of *Pu Ji Fang* 普济方 (c. 1406). Exposure to wind, heat and damp was thought to obstruct the flow of *qi* and Blood, and cause lichenification of the skin in children (夫小儿体有风热, 脾肺不利, 或湿邪搏于皮肤, 壅滞血气, 皮肤顽厚, 则变诸癣). Symptoms were reduced when cold (得寒则稍减), further highlighting heat as a key factor in the pathogenesis of atopic dermatitis.

Dysfunction of the Spleen and Lung was also implicated in the quote above from *Pu Ji Fang* 普济方. Dysfunction of the Spleen leads to formation of damp, which can either stagnate and turn to heat, or may combine with external pathogenic heat. In a passage from *Yang Ke Jie Jing* 疡科捷径 (c. 1831), both internal dampness-heat and external wind were considered to be involved in atopic dermatitis (外受风邪兼湿热).

The chronic nature of atopic dermatitis and treatment options were described in a passage from *Wai Ke Xin Fa Yao Jue* 外科心法要诀 (c. 1742). The itch associated with sores was attributed to Heart fire. This syndrome develops when syndromes of exterior deficiency syndrome and internal stagnation of fire pathogen co-exist, allowing external wind to invade the body surface and stir up fire. In this syndrome, the rash is red and shaped like millet; scratching increases itching. When recovery is prolonged, Blood is consumed, and the skin becomes dry and rough, like snake's skin. *Fang feng tong sheng san* 防风通圣散 with *zhi qiao* 枳壳 and *chan tui* 蝉蜕 can be taken orally. When severe itching at night disturbs sleep, *Xiao feng san* 消风散 can be taken and *Er wei ba du san* 二味拔毒散 can be used externally. If the disease duration is long and the skin is dry like snake's skin, *Zao jiao ku shen wan* 皂角苦参丸 should be taken often, and a mixture of two ounces of lard oil with one ounce *ku xing ren* 苦杏仁 applied externally is effective. (粟疮痒证属火生, 风邪乘皮起粟形, 风为火化能作痒, 通圣苦参及消风. [注] 凡诸疮作痒, 皆属心火. 火邪内郁, 表虚之人, 感受风邪, 袭入皮肤, 风遇火化作痒, 致起疮疡形如粟粒, 其色红, 搔之愈痒, 久而不瘥, 亦能消耗血液, 肤如蛇皮. 初服防风通圣散加枳壳, 蝉蜕, 血燥遇晚痒甚, 夜不寐者, 宜服消风散, 外敷二味拔毒散. 若年深日久, 肤如蛇皮者, 宜常服皂角苦参丸, 外用猪脂油二两, 苦杏仁一两捣泥, 抹之自效.)

Symptom Location

Seventy-five citations described the location of the atopic dermatitis, with 35 reporting symptoms in multiple locations. The most frequently reported location was the face, described in 18 citations.

Symptoms were grouped according to broad body location. The majority of symptoms were located on the head, face and neck (64 citations). Specific locations include the face, head, ear, eyebrows, cheek, nucha, nape/neck and mouth. Symptoms were less frequently seen on other body areas. Symptoms were on the lower limbs in 23 citations, covered the whole body in 16 citations and were on the torso in five citations, and one citation described symptoms on the upper limbs. Seventeen citations described symptoms as being located on the limbs, but did not specify whether these were upper or lower limbs. Eight citations specifically described symptoms in infants, and all eight described the location as being on the head, face or eyebrow.

Chinese Herbal Medicine

Of the 271 treatment citations, 268 described treatment with CHM. Among all CHM citations, it was not surprising to find that most citations included a description of skin rash (264 citations); itch was also frequently described (212 citations). Fewer citations described the rash appearing in flexural folds (77 citations), and whether the condition was chronic or relapsing (74 citations). In a subset of the CHM citations that were judged 'most likely' to be atopic dermatitis (at least three of the four characteristic symptoms), all citations described skin rash or skin dryness. Seventy-seven citations described itch, 51 described chronicity or the relapsing nature of the condition, and 42 citations described the location of the rash. From the classical CM literature, we can see that skin rash and itch were the main symptoms in possible cases of atopic dermatitis.

The earliest citation of the official term for atopic dermatitis, *si wan feng* 四弯风, was from the *Wai Ke Da Cheng* 外科大成 (c. 1665) in the Qing dynasty. The number of citations identified by this term was small compared to *jin yin chuang* 浸淫疮. While three of the 10 citations identified by *si wan feng* 四弯风 did not have sufficient information to permit judgment about their likelihood of being atopic dermatitis, the remaining seven were all judged 'most likely' to be atopic dermatitis. Five of these included descriptions of all four characteristic symptoms of atopic dermatitis: itch, skin rash, rash location matching conventional medical understanding, and chronicity/ recurrence of the condition.

Citations for CHM originated from 54 different books. Thirteen of these books included one citation considered 'possibly' related to atopic dermatitis, and 41 books included two or more citations. Three books yielded the highest number of included citations (22 citations each). These were *Wai Ke Xin Fa Yao Jue* 外科心法要诀 (c. 1742), *Tong Yuan Yi Shi (Wai Ke)* 彤园医书 (外科) (c. 1796) and the more recent *Wai Ke Bei Yao* 外科备要 (c. 1904). Other books which produced higher numbers of relevant citations included *Yi Xue Ru Men* 医学入门 (c. 1575; 15 citations), *Tai Ping Sheng Hui Fang* 太平圣惠方 (c. 992 CE; 13 citations), *Jiao Zhu Fu Ren Liang Fang* 校注妇人良方 (c. 1558; 10 citations) and Volumes 358–480 of *Pu Ji Fang* 普济方 (c. 1406; 10 citations).

Frequency of Treatment Citations by Dynasty

The majority of included citations were found in books from the Ming and Qing dynasties (87.1%) (Table 3.3). This is not surprising, as techniques for book publication advanced rapidly during both dynasties. The earliest citation describing treatment came from Ge Hong's 葛洪 *Zhou Hou Bei Ji Fang* 肘后备急方 (c. 363 CE). This citation was identified by the term *jin yin chuang* 浸淫疮. This term has

Table 3.3.   Dynastic Distribution of Treatment Citations

Dynasty	No. of Treatment Citations (%)
Before Tang dynasty (before 618)	2 (0.7)
Tang and Five dynasties (618–960)	2 (0.7)
Song and Jin dynasties (961–1271)	28 (10.3)
Yuan dynasty (1272–1368)	0 (0)
Ming dynasty (1369–1644)	90 (33.2)
Qing dynasty (1645–1911)	146 (53.9)
Minguo/Republic of China (1912–1949)	3 (1.1)
Total	**271 (100%)**

a long history of use, being used in books through to the Ming Guo period (*Xi Mi Chuan Jian Yan Fang* 溪秘传简验方, c. 1918).

The most recent citation was from He Limin's *Zeng Ding Tong Su Shang Han Lun* 增订通俗伤寒论 (c. 1929), was found by the term *xue feng chuang* 血风疮. All citations identified by the official Chinese term for atopic dermatitis, *si wan feng* 四弯风, were from the Qing dynasty, and all were judged to 'most likely' be atopic dermatitis based on characteristic descriptions. Citations from the Minguo/Republic of China were found with terms *xue feng chuang* 血风疮 and *tai xuan* 胎癣. The fact that *si wan feng* 四弯风 was not found in possible atopic dermatitis citations from the Minguo era was not surprising, as this term was not recognised as the official term until the publication of the *Guidelines for Chinese Medicine Diagnosis and Treatment* 中医病证诊断疗效标准 by the State Administration of Traditional Chinese Medicine in 1994.[7]

Treatment with Chinese Herbal Medicine

Of the 268 CHM treatment citations, 40 citations were pharmacopeia-type herb entries or single herb treatments, and 228 citations described multi-herb formulas. These citations were judged as either 'possible' cases of atopic dermatitis or 'most likely' cases of atopic dermatitis. Additional analysis of citations in the best pool of those judged 'most likely' to be atopic dermatitis was also conducted.

Most Frequent Formulas in 'Possible' Atopic Dermatitis Citations

Eighty-two CHM treatment citations did not specify the name of formulas. In some citations, formulas were described according to herb ingredients and/or the action of the formula for atopic dermatitis. For example, one citation from *Ying Er Lun* 婴儿论 (c. 1778) describes treatment with *Fang feng pai du yin* 防风排毒饮, which can be translated as '*Fang feng* 防风 detoxification drink.'

Named formulas in the citations were analysed to identify those that appeared most frequently in classical literature. Herb ingredients are presented for the earliest citation of the formula, as these were considered to be the basis from which future modifications were made. Where ingredients for formulas were not included in the citation, other sections of the same book were searched to identify ingredients of the formula. If these were unable to be located, the citation was noted as 'ingredients not specified.'

The majority of treatments were for topical use, with almost two thirds of the citations (167, 62.3%) describing topical application. Ninety-seven citations described oral administration (36.2%), and four suggested the formula be used both orally and topically (1.5%). The ten most frequently cited formulas can be found in Table 3.4. The most frequently used oral CHM formula was *Xiao feng san* 消风散

Table 3.4. Most Frequent Formulas in 'Possible' Atopic Dermatitis Citations

Formula Name	Herb Ingredients	Number of Citations (*n*)
Xiao feng san 消风散 (oral)	*Jing jie* 荆芥, *fang feng* 防风, *dang gui* 当归, *sheng di* 生地, *ku shen* 苦参, *cang zhu* 苍术, *chan tui* 蝉蜕, *hu ma ren* 胡麻仁, *niu bang zi* 牛蒡子, *shi gao* 石膏, *zhi mu* 知母, *gan cao* 甘草, *mu tong* 木通, *huang bai* 黄柏 and *niu xi* 牛膝. [This citation from *Wai Ke Zheng Zong* 外科正宗 (c. 1617) used *Xiao feng san* 消风散 plus *huang bai* 黄柏 and *niu xi* 牛膝].	13
Dang gui yin (*zi*) 当归饮(子) (oral)	*Dang gui* 当归, *bai shao* 白芍, *chuan xiong* 川芎, *sheng di huang* 生地黄, *bai ji li* 白蒺藜, *fang feng* 防风, *jing jie* 荆芥, *huang qi* 黄芪, *he shou wu* 何首乌, *gan cao* 甘草, *chai hu* 柴胡 and *shan zhi* 山栀. [This citation from *Nv Ke Cuo Yao* 女科撮要 (c. 1548) used *Dang gui yin* 当归饮 plus *chai hu* 柴胡 and *shan zhi* 山栀].	9
Gui pi tang 归脾汤 (oral)	*Ren shen* 人参, *bai zhu* 白术, *fu ling* 茯苓, *huang qi* 黄芪, *dang gui* 当归, *long yan rou* 龙眼肉, *yuan zhi* 远志, *suan zao ren* 酸枣仁, *mu xian* 木香 and *gan cao* 甘草. [*Nv Ke Cuo Yao* 女科撮要 (c. 1548)].	8

(Continued)

Table 3.4. (*Continued*)

Formula Name	Herb Ingredients	Number of Citations (*n*)
Run ji gao 润肌膏 (topical)	*Xiang you* 香油, *nai su you* 奶酥油, *dang gui* 当归, *zi cao* 紫草 and *huang la* 黄蜡. [*Wai Ke Xin Fa Yao Jue* 外科心法要诀 (c. 1742)].	8
Huang lian gao 黄连膏 (topical)	*Huang lian* 黄连, *dang gui wei* 当归尾, *sheng di* 生地, *huang bai* 黄柏, *jiang huang* 姜黄 and *huang la* 黄蜡. [*Wai Ke Xin Fa Yao Jue* 外科心法要诀 (c. 1742)].	5
Qing ha san 青蛤散 (topical)	*Bai jiao xiang* 白胶香, *ha fen* 蛤粉 and *qing dai* 青黛 [*Pu Ji Fang* 普济方 Volumes 358–480 (c. 1406)].	5
Xiao chai hu (*tang*) 小柴胡汤 (oral)	*Chai hu* 柴胡, *huang qin* 黄芩, *ban xia* 半夏, *ren shen* 人参, *gan cao* 甘草, *sheng jiang* 生姜, *da zao* 大枣, *shan zhi* 山栀 and *huang lian* 黄连. [This citation from *Nv Ke Cuo Yao* 女科撮要 (c. 1548) used *Xiao chai hu tang* 小柴胡汤 plus *shan zhi* 山栀 and *huang lian* 黄连].	5
Xiao yao san (*jia wei*) 加味逍遥散 (oral)	*Gan cao* 甘草, *dang gui* 当归, *shao yao* 芍药, *fu ling* 茯苓, *bai zhu* 白术, *chai hu* 柴胡, *mu dan pi* 牡丹皮 and *shan zhi* 山栀. [*Nv Ke Cuo Yao* 女科撮要 (c. 1548)].	5
Xiong huang jie du san 雄黄解毒散 (topical)	*Xiong huang* 雄黄, *han shui shi* 寒水石 and *bai fan* 白矾. [*Wai Ke Xin Fa Yao Jue* 外科心法要诀 (c. 1742)].	5
Zao jiao ku shen wan 皂角苦参丸 (oral)	*Ku shen* 苦参, *jing jie* 荆芥, *bai zhi* 白芷, *da feng zi rou* 大风子肉, *fang feng* 防风, *da zao jiao* 大皂角, *chuan xiong* 川芎, *dang gui* 当归, *he shou wu* 何首乌, *da hu ma* 大胡麻, *gou qi zi* 枸杞子, *niu bang zi* 牛蒡子, *wei ling xian* 威灵仙, *quan xie* 全蝎, *bai fu zi* 白附子, *ji li* 蒺藜, *du huo* 独活, *chuan niu xi* 川牛膝, *cao wu* 草乌, *cang zhu* 苍术, *lian qiao* 连翘, *tian ma* 天麻, *man jing zi* 蔓荆子, *qiang huo* 羌活, *qing feng teng* 青风藤, *gan cao* 甘草, *du zhong* 杜仲, *bai hua she* 白花蛇, *sha ren* 砂仁 and *ren shen* 人参. [*Wai Ke Xin Fa Yao Jue* 外科心法要诀 (c. 1742)].	5

Note: The use of some herbs may be restricted in some countries. Readers are advised to comply with relevant regulations.

(used in 13 citations), and the most frequently used topical CHM formula was *Run ji gao* 润肌膏 (used in eight citations).

Herb ingredients for some formulas varied over time, with 30 citations describing core formulas with additions. For example, the earliest citation of *Xiao feng san* 消风散 described *Xiao feng san* 消风散 plus *huang bai* 黃柏 and *niu xi* 牛膝 as a treatment for atopic dermatitis. This is interesting to note, as while modifying traditional formulas according to the patient's presentation is a usual part of clinical practice, citations do not normally state which herbs should be added or removed. In the 30 citations that detailed modifications, the most frequent additions were *shan zhi* 山栀 (11 citations), *huang lian* 黃连 (seven citations), *chai hu* 柴胡 (six citations), *sheng di huang* 生地黃 (five citations) and *shu di* 熟地 (four citations). Two herbs were removed from citations: *huang qi* 黃芪 (two citations) and *mu xiang* 木香 (one citation).

Most Frequent Herbs in 'Possible' Atopic Dermatitis Citations

There was a broad diversity in herbs, with a total of 231 different herbs described in CHM citations. The frequency was calculated separately for herbs that were for oral use and those for topical use. One hundred and twenty-three herbs were used orally. The number of herbs in oral CHM treatments varied from two to 30 herbs. The median number of herbs in oral CHM formulas was 11. The most frequently used herb was *gan cao* 甘草, described in 83 citations (Table 3.5). This is likely due to its action of harmonising the herbs in formulas. Other frequently used herbs included *dang gui* 当归 (72 citations), *fang feng* 防风 (40 citations), *bai shao* 白芍 (36 citations) and *sheng di huang* 生地黃 (36 citations).

While the number of citations for topical use was almost double the number for oral use, the diversity in topically used herbs was not as great. This is likely due to topical CHM formulas being less complex and involving fewer herbs. Some citations included topical use of single herbs, and the most complex treatments involved up to 11 herbs. The median number of herbs for topical CHM citations was two.

Table 3.5. Most Frequent Orally Used Herbs in 'Possible' Atopic Dermatitis Citations

Herb Name	Scientific Name	No. of Citations (*n*)
Gan cao 甘草	*Glycyrrhiza* spp	83
Dang gui 当归	*Angelica sinensis* (Oliv.) Diels	72
Fang feng 防风	*Saposhnikovia divaricata* (Turcz.) Schischk.	40
Bai shao 白芍	*Paeonia lactiflora* Pall.	36
Sheng di huang 生地黄	*Rehmannia glutinosa* Libosch.	36
Jing jie 荆芥	*Schizonepeta tenuifolia* Briq.	32
Ren shen 人参	*Panax ginseng* C. A. Mey.	31
Bai zhu 白术	*Atractylodes macrocephala* Koidz.	30
Chuan xiong 川芎	*Ligusticum chuangxiong* Hort.	28
Fu ling 茯苓	*Poria cocos* (Schw.) Wolf	28
Cang zhu 苍术	*Atractylodes* spp	26
Ku shen 苦参	*Sophora flavescens* Ait.	26
Niu bang zi 牛蒡子	*Arctium lappa* L.	26
Chai hu 柴胡	*Bupleurum* spp	24
Huang qi 黄芪	*Astragalus* spp	24
Sheng jiang 生姜	*Zingiber officinale* Rosc.	21
Bai ji li 白蒺藜	*Tribulus terrestris* L.	20
Hu ma ren 胡麻仁	*Lespedeza dunnii* Schindle	20
Shu di huang 熟地黄	*Rehmannia glutinosa* Libosch.	20

Note: The use of some herbs may be restricted in some countries. Readers are advised to comply with relevant regulations.

One hundred and fifty-six topically used herbs were identified in citations 'possibly' related to atopic dermatitis. The most frequently used herbs for topical application included *huang bai* 黄柏 (29 citations), *qing fen* 轻粉 (29 citations), *bai fan* 白矾 (26 citations) and *ma you* 麻油 (23 citations) (Table 3.6). Several of the frequently used herbs used topically are likely to be excipients with no therapeutic effect. For example, *ma you* 麻油 is typically used to bind the formula together to make a paste for topical application. Whilst these herbs do not have therapeutic actions, their inclusion is nevertheless

Table 3.6. Most Frequent Topically Used Herbs in 'Possible' Atopic Dermatitis Citations

Herb Name	Scientific Name	No. of Citations (*n*)
Huang bai 黄柏	*Phellodendron chinense* Schneid.	29
Qing fen 轻粉	Mercurous chloride	29
Bai fan 白矾	Potassium aluminium sulfate	26
Ma you 麻油	Sesame oil	23
Dang gui 当归	*Angelica sinensis* (Oliv.) Diels	18
Xiong huang 雄黄	Arsenic disulfide	18
Huang la 黄蜡	Beeswax	16
Huang lian 黄连	*Coptis* spp	15
Gan cao 甘草	*Glycyrrhiza* spp	11
Hu fen 胡粉	Lead powder	9
Liu huang 硫黄	Sulfur	9
Huang dan 黄丹	Lead oxide	8
Ma chi xian 马齿苋	*Portulaca oleracea* L.	8
Zi cao 紫草	*Arnebia* spp	8
Han shui shi 寒水石	Calcite/Gypsum rubrum	7
Ji guan xue 鸡冠血	Coxcomb blood	7
Ji yu 鲫鱼	Carassius auratus	7
Zhu zhi 猪脂	Pig fat	7

Note: The use of some herbs may be restricted in some countries. Readers are advised to comply with relevant regulations.

important as they provide insight into how topical CHM formulations were prepared.

Four citations described the use of a CHM treatment orally and topically, although only two citations named the formula and only one described the herbs. Many of the herbs prescribed for both oral and topical use were among the most frequently used oral herbs e.g. *dang gui* 当归, *bai shao* 白芍 and *gan cao* 甘草.

Most Frequent Formulas in 'Most Likely' Atopic Dermatitis Citations

Based on descriptions of characteristic symptoms, 80 citations were judged 'most likely' to be related to atopic dermatitis. As found in the total pool, topical treatment with CHM was seen more frequently than oral CHM. Fifty-one citations described topical CHM formulas, and 27 described oral CHM formulas. Two citations suggested the formula be used orally and topically; however, the formula was not named, nor were ingredients listed. The findings for 'most likely' atopic dermatitis citations were similar to the overall pool in terms of the formulas used. *Xiao feng san* 消风散 was the most frequently used oral formula (eight citations) and *Run ji gao* 润肌膏 the most frequently cited topical formula (seven citations) (Table 3.7).

Eleven of the 13 most frequently used citations were from the book *Wai Ke Xin Fa Yao Jue* 外科心法要诀 (c. 1742). *Wai Ke Xin Fa Yao Jue* 外科心法要诀 is a part of the compilation *Yi Zong Jin Jian* 医宗金鉴 (*Golden Mirror of Orthodox Medicine*), a 90-volume collection used as a textbook by the Imperial Medical School during the Qing dynasty.[14] As described earlier, this book was one of the three that produced the highest number of citations.

Two oral formulas were used frequently in both the 'possible' and 'most likely' pools: *Xiao feng san* 消风散 and *Zao jiao ku shen wan* 皂角苦参丸. Interestingly, several of the orally used formulas that were frequently seen in 'possible' atopic dermatitis citations were not found in the 'most likely' atopic dermatitis citations. For example, the formulas *Dang gui yin zi* 当归饮子, *Gui pi tang* 归脾汤, *Xiao chai hu tang* 小柴胡汤 and *Xiao yao san* 逍遥散 were among the most frequently used formulas in the total pool, but were not described in 'most likely' atopic dermatitis citations. Of the 28 citations that used these four formulas, 25 citations were identified by the term '*xue feng chuang* 血风疮.' This term can be translated as 'Blood-wind sores.' It would seem logical that formulas that tonify Blood and dispel wind, such as *Dang gui yin zi* 当归饮子, would be used for this condition. However, this term also identified 23 of the 80 'most likely' atopic dermatitis citations that were treated by a wide variety of other oral

Table 3.7.   Most Frequent Formulas in 'Most Likely' Atopic Dermatitis Citations

Formula Name	Herb Ingredients	No. of Citations (*n*)
Xiao feng san 消风散 (oral)	*Jing jie* 荆芥, *fang feng* 防风, *dang gui* 当归, *sheng di* 生地, *ku shen* 苦参, *cang zhu* 苍术, *chan tui* 蝉蜕, *hu ma ren* 胡麻仁, *niu bang zi* 牛蒡子, *shi gao* 石膏, *zhi mu* 知母, *gan cao* 甘草, *mu tong* 木通, *huang bai* 黄柏 and *niu xi* 牛膝. [This citation from *Wai Ke Zheng Zong* 外科正宗 (c. 1617) used *Xiao feng san* 消风散 with *huang bai* 黄柏 and *niu xi* 牛膝.]	8
Run ji gao 润肌膏 (topical)	*Xiang you* 香油, *nai su you* 奶酥油, *dang gui* 当归, *zi cao* 紫草 and *huang la* 黄蜡. [*Wai Ke Xin Fa Yao Jue* 外科心法要诀 (c. 1742)].	7
Zao jiao ku shen wan 皂角苦参丸 (oral)	*Ku shen* 苦参, *jing jie* 荆芥, *bai zhi* 白芷, *da feng zi rou* 大风子肉, *fang feng* 防风, *da zao jiao* 大皂角, *chuan xiong* 川芎, *dang gui* 当归, *he shou wu* 何首乌, *da hu ma* 大胡麻, *gou qi zi* 枸杞子, *niu bang zi* 牛蒡子, *wei ling xian* 威灵仙, *quan xie* 全蝎, *bai fu zi* 白附子, *ji li* 蒺藜, *du huo* 独活, *chuan niu xi* 川牛膝, *cao wu* 草乌, *cang zhu* 苍术, *lian qiao* 连翘, *tian ma* 天麻, *man jing zi* 蔓荆子, *qiang huo* 羌活, *qing feng teng* 青风藤, *gan cao* 甘草, *du zhong* 杜仲, *bai hua she* 白花蛇, *sha ren* 砂仁 and *ren shen* 人参. [*Wai Ke Xin Fa Yao Jue* 外科心法要诀 (c. 1742)].	4
Di huang yin 地黄饮 (oral)	*Sheng di* 生地, *shu di* 熟地, *he shou wu* 何首乌, *dang gui* 当归, *dan pi* 丹皮, *hei can* 黑参, *bai ji li* 白蒺藜, *jiang can* 僵蚕, *hong hua* 红花 and *gan cao* 甘草. [*Wai Ke Xin Fa Yao Jue* 外科心法要诀 (c. 1742)].	3
Er wei ba du san 二味拔毒散 (topical)	*Xiong huang* 雄黄 and *bai fan* 白矾. (*Wai Ke Xin Fa Yao Jue* 外科心法要诀 (c. 1742)].	3

(Continued)

Table 3.7.   (***Continued***)

Formula Name	Herb Ingredients	No. of Citations (*n*)
Fang feng tong sheng san 防风通圣散 (oral)	*Fang feng* 防风, *dang gui* 当归, *bai shao* 白芍, *mang xiao* 芒硝, *da huang* 大黄, *lian qiao* 连翘, *jie geng* 桔梗, *chuan xiong* 川芎, *shi gao* 石膏, *huang qin* 黄芩, *bo he* 薄荷, *ma huang* 麻黄, *hua shi* 滑石, *jing jie* 荆芥, *bai zhu* 白术, *shan zhi zi* 山栀子, *gan cao* 甘草, *zhi ke* 枳壳 and *chan tui* 蝉蜕. [*Wai Ke Xin Fa Yao Jue* 外科心法要诀 (c. 1742)].	3
Huang lian gao 黄连膏 (topical)	*Huang lian* 黄连, *dang gui wei* 当归尾, *sheng di* 生地, *huang bai* 黄柏, *jiang huang* 姜黄 and *huang la* 黄蜡. [*Wai Ke Xin Fa Yao Jue* 外科心法要诀 (c. 1742)].	3
Jie du xiong huang san 解毒雄黄散 (topical)	*Xiong huang* 雄黄 and *liu huang* 硫黄. [*Wai Ke Zheng Zhong* 外科正宗 (c. 1617)].	3
San miao san 三妙散 (topical)	*Bin lang* 槟榔, *cang zhu* 苍术 and *huang bai* 黄柏. [*Wai Ke Xin Fa Yao Jue* 外科心法要诀 (c. 1742)].	3
Wu fu hua du dan 五福化毒丹 (oral)	*Hei shen* 黑参, *chi fu ling* 赤茯苓, *jie geng* 桔梗, *ya xiao* 牙硝, *qing dai* 青黛, *huang lian* 黄连, *long dan cao* 龙胆草, *gan cao* 甘草, *ren shen* 人参, *zhu sha* 朱砂 and *bing pian* 冰片. [*Wai Ke Xin Fa Yao Jue* 外科心法要诀 (c. 1742)].	3
Wu yun gao 乌云膏 (topical)	*Song xiang mo* 松香末, *liu huang* 硫黄 and *xiang you* 香油. (*Wai Ke Xin Fa Yao Jue* 外科心法要诀 (c. 1742)].	3
Xiao feng dao chi tang 消风导赤汤 (oral)	*Shen di* 生地, *chi shao* 赤芍, *niu bang zi* 牛蒡子, *bai xian pi* 白鲜皮, *yin hua* 银花, *bo he* 薄荷, *mu tong* 木通, *huang lian* 黄连 and *gan cao* 甘草. [*Wai Ke Xin Fa Yao Jue* 外科心法要诀 (c. 1742)].	3
Xiong huang jie du san 雄黄解毒散 (topical)	*Xiong huang* 雄黄, *han shui shi* 寒水石 and *bai fan* 白矾. (*Wai Ke Xin Fa Yao Jue* 外科心法要诀 (c. 1742)].	3

and topical CHM formulas. So, the absence of these four formulas cannot be explained by the search term. Another common feature of the 28 citations that used these four formulas was that they all included descriptions of itch and skin rash, but no mention of the rash location or chronicity/relapse. It is possible that these formulas were used to treat other skin conditions that presented with itch and skin rash but were not atopic dermatitis. When the clinical effect with CHM is suboptimal, clinicians could choose one of these four formulas according to syndrome differentiation.

Most Frequent Herbs in 'Most Likely' Atopic Dermatitis Citations

As was seen in frequently used herbs in 'possible' atopic dermatitis citations, there was great diversity in herb ingredients. Seventy-seven different herbs were used in the 80 citations, and formulas varied in size from nine to 30 herbs. The median number of herbs in 'most likely' atopic dermatitis citations was 13. The herbs frequently used in most likely atopic dermatitis citations were similar to those seen in 'possible' atopic dermatitis citations. In fact, the three most common herbs in both pools were *gan cao* 甘草, *dang gui* 当归 and *fang feng* 防风 (Table 3.8).

One herb frequently seen in 'possible' atopic dermatitis citations that was not found in 'most likely' citations was *chai hu* 柴胡. The 'possible' atopic dermatitis citations that included *chai hu* 柴胡 were all found with the term *xue feng chuang* 血风疮. However, this finding is unlikely to be relevant, as several of the best citations were found using *xue feng chuang* 血风疮. Indeed, none of the formulas recommended in contemporary guidelines described in Chapter 2 include *chai hu* 柴胡. Based on preference, clinical experience or syndrome differentiation, other herbs may have been used in preference to *chai hu* 柴胡.

There was less diversity in the herbs for topical use than for oral use. Fifty-seven different herbs were described in the 51 citations. As was seen in the total pool, topical treatments were simpler. The number of herb ingredients ranged from one to 11 herbs, and the median number of herbs included in topical treatments was three.

Table 3.8.   Most Frequent Orally Used Herbs in 'Most Likely' Atopic Dermatitis Citations

Herb Name	Scientific Name	No. of Citations (*n*)
Gan cao 甘草	*Glycyrrhiza* spp	26
Dang gui 当归	*Angelica sinensis* (Oliv.) Diels	20
Fang feng 防风	*Saposhnikovia divaricata* (Turcz.) Schischk.	16
Jing jie 荆芥	*Schizonepeta tenuifolia* Briq.	15
Niu bang zi 牛蒡子	*Arctium lappa* L.	15
Sheng di huang 生地黄	*Rehmannia glutinosa* Libosch.	13
Cang zhu 苍术	*Atractylodes* spp	12
Hu ma ren 胡麻仁	*Lespedeza dunnii* Schindle	12
Ku shen 苦参	*Sophora flavescens* Ait.	12
Shi gao 石膏	Hydrated calcium sulfate	11
Chan tui 蝉蜕	*Cryptotympana pustulata* Fabricius	10
Jie geng 桔梗	*Platycodon grandiflorum* (Jacq.) A. DC.	10
Chuan xiong 川芎	*Ligusticum chuangxiong* Hort.	9
Zhi mu 知母	*Anemarrhena asphodeloides* Bge.	8
Bai ji li 白蒺藜	*Tribulus terrestris* L.	7
He shou wu 何首乌	*Polygonum multiflorum* Thunb.	7
Lian qiao 连翘	*Forsythia suspensa* (Thunb.) Vahl	7
Mu tong 木通	*Akebia* spp	7
Xuan shen 玄参	*Scrophularia ningpoensis* Hemsl.	7

Note: The use of some herbs may be restricted in some countries. Readers are advised to comply with relevant regulations.

Ma you 麻油 was the most frequently used herb, described in 15 citations (Table 3.9). The topical herbs frequently used in the 'most likely' atopic dermatitis were mostly consistent with the total pool. Some of the herbs included in Table 3.9 were not in the top 20 most frequently used herbs in the total pool. This is likely to be related to the smaller subset of citations judged 'most likely' to be atopic dermatitis, and overall lower frequency of herbs in this subset.

Two citations judged 'most likely' to be atopic dermatitis described treatments which should be applied orally and topically.

Table 3.9.   Most Frequent Topically Used Herbs in 'Most Likely' Atopic Dermatitis Citations

Herb Name	Scientific Name	No. of Citations (*n*)
Ma you 麻油	Sesame oil	15
Dang gui 当归	*Angelica sinensis* (Oliv.) Diels	12
Huang bai 黄柏	*Phellodendron chinense* Schneid.	10
Huang la 黄蜡	Beeswax	10
Bai fan 白矾	Potassium aluminium sulfate	9
Xiong huang 雄黄	Arsenic disulfide	9
Zi cao 紫草	*Arnebia* spp	7
Zhu zhi 猪脂	Pig fat	6
Liu huang 硫黄	Sulfur	6
Cang zhu 苍术	*Atractylodes* spp	5
Qing fen 轻粉	Mercurous chloride	5
Han shui shi 寒水石	Calcite/Gypsum rubrum	4
Huang lian 黄连	*Coptis* spp	4
Jiang huang 姜黄	*Curcuma longa* L.	4
Ren ru zhi 人乳汁	Human milk	4
Bing lan 槟榔	*Areca catechu* L.	3
Da huang 大黄	*Rheum* spp	3
Da mai 大麦	*Hordeum vulgare* L.	3
Gan cao 甘草	*Glycyrrhiza* spp	3
Sheng di 生地	*Rehmannia glutinosa* Libosch.	3
Song xiang mo 松香末	*Pinus tabulaeformix* Carr.	3

Note: The use of some herbs may be restricted in some countries. Readers are advised to comply with relevant regulations.

No details were available for the formula name, nor were herb ingredients described.

Other Chinese Medicine Therapies

Three citations described treatments other than CHM. All citations were from books published in the Ming and Qing dynasties, and all were identified by the term *xue feng chuang* 血风疮. The earliest citation came from *Wai Ke Zhen Zong* 外科正宗 (c. 1617), and was judged most likely to relate to atopic dermatitis. It described a technique of pricking the skin to clear Blood stasis. Another citation from *Wu Shi Yi Fang Hui Bian* 吴氏医方汇编 (c. 1823) described the same technique, although there was less certainty of whether the citation related to atopic dermatitis. The third citation was found in the book *Yang Ke Xin De Ji* 疡科心得集 (c. 1805), and was found to be 'most likely' atopic dermatitis. This citation described the use of acupuncture (*bian fa* 砭法), but no further details were provided.

Classical Literature in Perspective

Atopic dermatitis has been described throughout classical CM literature, appearing in 54 books included in the ZHYD. The term that identified the greatest number of citations, *jin yin chuang* 浸淫疮, has been synonymous with atopic dermatitis from the pre-Tang dynasty through to the Minguo/Republic of China. The same can be said of the second-most productive term: *xue feng chuang* 血风疮. This term was identified in *Hua Tuo Shen Fang* 华佗神方 from the Tang and Five dynasties (c. 682), and the most recent citation was from *Zeng Ding Tong Su Shang Han Lun* 增订通俗伤寒论 (c. 1929). Fewer citations were found with the term *si wan feng* 四弯风, which was not surprising given this is a more modern term.

The syndromes described in classical literature were similar to those described in contemporary guidelines (see Chapter 2), and those identified in classical literature research by Huang *et al.* (2011).[2] Chinese medicine physicians understood atopic dermatitis to be a hereditary disease. They also understood that atopic dermatitis resulted from both internal and external causes, often in concert. The interplay between internal and external causes was highlighted in a passage from *Yang Ke Jie Jing* 疡科捷径. Liang, cited in Radikoff, Cohen and Scheinfeld (2014),[15] has suggested this concept can also be seen in the conventional medical 'inside-out' and 'outside-in' hypotheses (see Chapter 1). Thus, some parallels can be seen in conventional and CM understanding of atopic dermatitis.

The nature of symptoms described in citations in this review differed from those described by Huang *et al.* (2011).[2] The proportion of symptoms affecting the head and face was higher in this research (64 citations, 85.3% versus 26 citations, 53.1%), and was lower for symptoms affecting the entire body (16 citations, 21.3% versus 23 citations, 46.9%); results were similar for symptoms affecting the lower legs (23 citations, 30.6% versus 14 citations, 28.6%). This could be due to several factors. Firstly, a larger number of citations were included in this research (271 citations in total; 75 citations described symptoms), compared with 71 citations (49 of which described symptoms) in the research by Huang *et al.*[2] Secondly, differences in the books searched may have produced different results. More than 1,100 books of various specialties are included in the ZHYD, while Huang *et al.*[2] selected 24 key books related to dermatology. As the terms used by Huang *et al.*[2] were all included in this review, it seems likely that some books used in their research are not included in the ZHYD, particularly considering the number of citations with symptoms affecting the entire body was higher in their research. As the 24 books used in Huang *et al.*'s research were not described in the article, we were unable to determine whether this is the case. The third possible explanation is that citations included in Huang *et al.*'s research were excluded from this review. Comparison between the findings of this research and those of Tan (2014)[3] was not possible due to differences in the way data were presented.

The description of symptoms in the included citations appears to match the contemporary understanding of atopic dermatitis. Citations describing a rash in infants described symptoms appearing on the head, face or eyebrows; Eichenfield *et al.* (2014)[16] suggest that infants and children typically have head, neck and extensor surface involvement of the arms and legs. Eichenfield *et al.*[16] also suggest that adolescents and adults typically present with flexural dermatitis on the elbow or knee. For many of the citations included in this review, it was not possible to determine whether the case was of a child or adult. Based on typical presentation, it may be possible that citations found by the term *si wan feng* 四弯风 described atopic dermatitis in adolescents and adults, as all citations of *si wan feng* 四弯风 described leg involvement.

The majority of treatment citations related to CHM, and external treatments were favoured. The most frequently reported topical formula in citations 'most likely' to be atopic dermatitis was *Run ji gao* 润肌膏, and the most common oral formula was *Xiao feng san* 消风散. The earliest citation of *Xiao feng san* 消风散 was from the Qing dynasty, and it continues to be used in contemporary practice (see Chapter 2). *Run ji gao* 润肌膏 was not included as a treatment option in guidelines reviewed in Chapter 2, and the reasons for this are unclear. Two other CHM formulas recommended in guidelines in Chapter 2 were found in classical literature: *Dang gui yin zi* 当归饮子 and *Fang feng tong sheng wan (san)* 防风通圣散(散).

Some differences were noted between the findings of this review and those of previous research. Compared with our findings for the 'possible' atopic dermatitis pool, Huang *et al.*[2] reported a higher frequency of *Jie du xiong huang san* 解毒雄黄散 (seven citations versus three citations) and *Wen ge san* 文蛤散 (five citations versus two citations), and a lower frequency of *Run ji gao* 润肤肌膏 (four citations versus eight citations). As suggested above, the different resources used to identify classical literature citations of atopic dermatitis is likely to be the reason for such differences. The findings of Tan[3] were similar, which was not surprising given that the same database was used.

Differences were observed in herb ingredients compared with previous research, with Tan[3] reporting higher frequencies of herbs used topically and lower frequency of orally used herbs. For example, *qing fen* 轻粉 was found in 49 citations in Tan's research and in 29 citations in this review. Similar findings were seen for the excipients *ma you* 麻油 and *zhu zhi* 猪脂. For orally used herbs, the differences in herb frequencies were more pronounced. *Gan cao* 甘草 was found in 83 citations in this research, compared with 22 citations in Tan's research. This trend was also evident for *dang gui* 当归 (72 citations versus 13 citations), *fang feng* 防风 (40 citations versus 11 citations) and *niu bang zi* 牛蒡子 (26 citations versus 11 citations). There are several possible reasons for the observed differences. Firstly, the number of search terms and subsequently included citations in the research by Tan was greater than in this research. Second, one of the terms used by Tan, *gan xuan* 干癣, may be more likely to identify other types of eczema or other skin conditions, as it is one of the current Chinese terms for psoriasis or tinea.[3] Finally, different selection criteria were used in Tan's study and this one, which may have contributed to the different results seen.

Chinese herbal medicine was the main treatment method used to treat 'possible' cases of atopic dermatitis, with very few citations found that employed other methods. One citation described the use of acupuncture (*bian fa* 砭法), but it did not describe which acupuncture points or meridians should be used. Acupuncture is recommended in current guidelines included in Chapter 2, with a focus on treating deficiency and expelling external pathogens. Two citations described pricking the skin, although the site of application was not mentioned. This technique was not recommended in guidelines included in Chapter 2, and its clinical use remains uncertain.

The findings of this research have several limitations. Terminology and language in classical CM literature have changed over time and their meanings rely on interpretation. It is possible that the original meaning has been misunderstood, which may have resulted in potentially relevant citations being excluded and potentially irrelevant citations being included. The selection of search terms for use ultimately determines which citations are considered for inclusion, and this may have biased the results. In addition, inclusion criteria were applied to identify potentially relevant citations. It is possible that descriptions of atopic dermatitis were excluded where detailed descriptions of the symptoms were lacking. While inclusion criteria were used, assessment still required reading, interpretation and judgment, and it is possible that this process excluded citations which may have been relevant.

Assessment of the frequency of oral and topical CHM formulas was based on formula name. It is possible that formulas with the same herb ingredients but different names existed in the dataset. Due to the difficulties in assessing the similarity of formulas based on ingredients, and formulas with modifications that have been renamed, it was not possible to make an assessment of which formulas were similar enough to be merged for frequency analysis. This may result in an underestimation of formula frequency. Finally, the appearance of atopic dermatitis differs between the acute and chronic stages. Researchers who read and selected citations for inclusion are qualified dermatologists with clinical experience. As data mining of the classical literature requires reading, interpretation and judgment, it is possible that human error may have resulted in a bias in the selection of citations.

Overall, the findings from evaluation of the classical literature show a strong emphasis of the management of atopic dermatitis with CHM, and a particular preference for topical CHM treatments. These findings can act as a guide for clinicians when selecting treatment, and clinicians should be encouraged to locate the clinical evidence to support their use.

References

1. Needham J, Lu G, Sivin N. (2000) *Science and Civilisation in China. Vol 5, Part VI: Medicine.* Cambridge University Press, Cambridge, UK.

2. 黄楚君, 蔡坚雄, 刘炽, *et al.* (2011) 特应性皮炎古籍文献的内容评析. 时珍国医国药 **22**(6): 1492–1494.

3. Tan HY. (2014) *Evaluation of the Safety and Efficacy of Chinese Medicine Treatment in the Management of Atopic Dermatitis.* RMIT University, Melbourne.

4. Hu R. (2000) *Encyclopedia of Traditional Chinese Medicine.* Hunan Electronic and Audio-Visual Publishing House, Changsha.

5. May B, Lu C, Xue C. (2012) Collections of traditional Chinese medical literature as resources for systematic searches. *J Altern Complement Med* **18**(12): 1101–1107.

6. May B, Lu Y, Lu C, *et al.* (2013) Systematic assessment of the representativeness of published collections of the traditional literature on Chinese Medicine. *J Altern Complement Med* **19**(5): 403–409.

7. 国家中医药管理局. (1994) 中医病证诊断疗效标准. 南京: 南京大学出版社.

8. 刘炽. (2015) 中医皮肤病症状鉴别诊断与治疗. 北京: 科学技术出版社.

9. 顾伯华. (1987) 中医外科学. 北京: 人民卫生出版社.

10. 赵尚华. (2002) 中医外科学. 北京: 人民卫生出版社.

11. Hinz D, Bauer M, Roder S, *et al.* (2012) Cord blood Tregs with stable FOXP3 expression are influenced by prenatal environment

and associated with atopic dermatitis at the age of one year. *Allergy* **67**(3): 380–389.

12. Nutten S. (2015) Atopic dermatitis: Global epidemiology and risk factors. *Ann Nutr Metab* **66** (Suppl 1): 8–16.

13. Lyttleton J. (2004) *Treatment of Infertility with Chinese Medicine.* Churchill Livingstone, Edinburgh, UK.

14. Helme M, Damone B, Brand E. (Shen Yu, trans.) (2005) *A Heart Approach to Gynecology: Essentials in Verse.* Paradigm Publications, Taos, New Mexico.

15. Radikoff D, Cohen SR, Scheinfeld N. (2014) *Atopic Dermatitis and Eczematous Disorders.* CRC Press, London.

16. Eichenfield LF, Tom WL, Chamlin SL, *et al.* (2014) Guidelines of care for the management of atopic dermatitis: Section 1. Diagnosis and assessment of atopic dermatitis. *J Am Acad Dermatol* **70**(2): 338–351.

4

Methods for Evaluating Clinical Evidence

OVERVIEW

Clinical studies of Chinese medicine interventions for atopic dermatitis were identified through searching electronic databases. Studies were assessed against eligibility criteria, and a review was conducted using standardised methods. This chapter describes the methods used to evaluate the efficacy and safety of Chinese medicine treatments for atopic dermatitis.

Introduction

Chinese medicine (CM) has been used for atopic dermatitis for many years. Contemporary literature describes treatments including Chinese herbal medicine (CHM) formulas and acupuncture therapies, many of which have their origins in the classical literature. Several systematic reviews have evaluated the efficacy and safety of CM treatments for atopic dermatitis. These reviews have been summarised in the relevant chapters.

This chapter will describe the methods used to identify and evaluate CM interventions for atopic dermatitis in clinical studies. Efficacy and safety will be examined in controlled clinical trials (CCTs). Interventions have been categorised as follows:

- CHM (Chapter 5).
- Acupuncture and related therapies (Chapter 7).
- Other CM therapies (Chapter 7).
- Combination CM therapies (Chapter 8).

Table 4.1.   Chinese Medicine Interventions Included in Clinical Evidence Evaluation

Category	Intervention
Chinese herbal medicines	Oral or topical.
Acupuncture and related therapies	Acupuncture, acupressure, ear acupuncture, ear acupressure, electroacupuncture, laser acupuncture, moxibustion, transcutaneous electrical nerve stimulation (TENS) and plum-blossom needle acupuncture.
Other Chinese medicine therapies	*Tuina* 推拿 (Chinese massage), cupping, *qigong* therapy 气功, *taichi* therapy 太極 and Chinese medicine diet therapy.
Combination Chinese medicine	Combination therapies are defined as two or more Chinese medicine interventions from different categories administered together e.g. Chinese herbal medicine plus acupuncture, or Chinese herbal medicine plus *qigong* therapy 气功.

An expert group of researchers identified and assessed references to clinical studies. Randomised controlled trials (RCTs), non-randomised controlled trials (CCTs) and non-controlled studies were evaluated in detail. Both randomised and non-randomised controlled trials were evaluated using the same approach, but the findings from these two types of studies have been described separately. Evidence from non-controlled studies is more difficult to evaluate, therefore the approach was taken to describe the characteristics of the study, details of the intervention and any adverse events. References to included studies are indicated by a letter followed by a number. Studies of CHM are indicated by a 'H' e.g. H1; studies of acupuncture and related therapies indicated by an 'A' e.g. A1; studies of other CM therapies indicated by an 'O' e.g. O1; and studies of combinations of CM therapies (see Table 4.1) indicated by a 'C' e.g. C1.

Search Strategy

Evidence was searched in English- and Chinese-language databases, and the methods followed the Cochrane Handbook of Systematic Reviews.[1] English-language databases included PubMed, Excerpta

Medica Database (Embase), Cumulative Index of Nursing and Allied Health Literature (CINAHL), Cochrane Central Register of Controlled Trials (CENTRAL) including the Cochrane Library, and Allied and Complementary Medicine Database (AMED). Chinese-language databases included China BioMedical Literature (CBM), China National Knowledge Infrastructure (CNKI), Chongqing VIP (CQVIP) and Wanfang. Databases were searched from inception to January 2017. No restrictions were applied. Search terms were mapped to controlled vocabulary (where applicable), in addition to being searched as keywords.

To conduct a comprehensive search of the literature, searches were run according to the study design (reviews, controlled trials and non-controlled studies). This was done for each of the three intervention types (CHM, acupuncture and related therapies, and other CM therapies) resulting in nine searches in each of the nine databases:

1. Reviews of CHM.
2. Controlled trials of CHM (randomised and non-randomised).
3. Non-controlled studies of CHM.
4. Reviews of acupuncture and related therapies.
5. Controlled trials of acupuncture and related therapies (randomised and non-randomised).
6. Non-controlled studies of acupuncture and related therapies.
7. Reviews of other CM therapies.
8. Controlled trials of other CM therapies (randomised and non-randomised).
9. Non-controlled studies of other CM therapies.

Studies of combination CM therapies were identified through the above searches. In addition to electronic databases, reference lists of systematic reviews and included studies were searched for additional publications. Clinical trial registries were searched to identify clinical trials which were ongoing or complete. The searched trial registries included the Australian New Zealand Clinical Trial Registry (ANZCTR), the Chinese Clinical Trial Registry (ChiCTR), the European Union Clinical Trials Register (EU-CTR) and the United States of America

National Institutes of Health register (ClinicalTrials.gov). If required, trial investigators were contacted to obtain further information. Trial investigators were contacted by email or telephone and were followed up after two weeks if no reply was received. Where no response was received after one month, any unknown information was marked as not available.

Inclusion Criteria

- Participants: People with atopic dermatitis or atopic eczema according to physician diagnosis, United Kingdom Working Party's diagnostic criteria (1994),[2] Hanifin and Rajka diagnostic criteria (1980)[3] or other diagnostic criteria.
- Interventions: Chinese medicine interventions (Table 4.1).
- Comparators: No treatment or waitlist control, sham/placebo or conventional medicines recommended in clinical practice guidelines.[4–10]
- Outcome measures: Studies reported at least one of the pre-specified outcome measures (Table 4.2).

Exclusion Criteria

- Participants: People with non-atopic dermatitis or infantile eczema.
- Interventions: Any intervention other than those considered to be CM.
- Comparators: Chinese medicine, treatments other than those recommended in clinical practice guidelines.
- Outcome measures: Therapeutic effective rate using criteria or descriptions other than those outlined in Table 4.2.

Outcomes

Existing resources, including the Harmonizing Outcome Measures for Eczema (HOME) consensus,[11] were consulted in determining outcomes for inclusion. Selected outcomes were confirmed by clinical experts and pre-specified prior to study selection. Outcomes were

Table 4.2.   Pre-specified Outcomes

Outcome Categories	Outcome Measures	Scoring
Clinician-reported eczema signs	1. EASI[12]	0 to 72, lower is better
	2. SCORAD[13]	0 to 103, lower is better
	3. SASSAD[14]	0 to 108, lower is better
	4. TIS[15]	0 to 9, lower is better
	5. IGA	0 to 5,* lower is better
	6. Scoring system of Rajka and Langeland[16]	3 to 9, lower is better
	7. Skin barrier function (TEWL)	NA
	8. Other clinician-reported signs	NA
Patient-reported eczema symptoms	1. POEM[17]	0 to 28, lower is better
	2. PO-SCORAD[18]	0 to 103, lower is better
	3. SA-EASI[19]	0 to 96, lower is better
	4. ADQ[20]	0 to 70, lower is better
	5. NESS[21]	3 to 15, lower is better
	6. ISS[22]	0 to 21, lower is better
	7. Other patient-reported symptoms e.g. sleep loss	NA
Long-term control	1. Relapse	Count, lower is better
	2. Time to recurrence	Length of time
	3. Other measures of long-term control	NA
Health-related quality of life	1. QoLIAD[23]	0–25 points, lower is better
	2. Skindex-29[24]	0–100 points, lower is better
	3. DLQI[25]	0 to 30, lower is better
	4. CDLQI[26]	0 to 30, lower is better
	5. SF36[27]	0–100 points per domain, higher is better
	6. EQ-5D[28]	See text
Effective rate	Effective rate[29,30]	Number of cases, higher is better
Adverse events	Number and type of adverse events	

*Variation exists in nomenclature, scale structure and score range for IGA; the most frequently used in RCTs is a six-point scale.[31]

Abbreviations: ADQ, Atopic Dermatitis Quickscore; CDLQI, Children's Dermatology Life Quality Index; DLQI, Dermatology Life Quality Index; EASI, Eczema Area Severity Index; EQ-5D, EuroQoL-5 Dimensions questionnaire; IGA, Investigator's Global Assessment; ISS, Itch Severity Scale; NA, not available; NESS, Nottingham Eczema Severity Score; PO-SCORAD, Patient-oriented SCOring Atopic Dermatitis Index; POEM, Patient-oriented Eczema Measure; QoLIAD, Quality of Life Index for Atopic Dermatitis; SA-EASI, Self-administered Eczema Area and Severity Index; SASSAD, Six Area, Six Sign Atopic Dermatitis; SCORAD, SCOring Atopic Dermatitis Index; SF36, Medical Outcome Study Short Form 36-item questionnaire; TEWL, transepidermal water loss; TIS, Three-item Severity score.

grouped into six categories: (1) clinician-reported eczema signs; (2) patient-reported eczema symptoms; (3) long-term control; (4) health-related quality of life; (5) therapeutic effective rate and (6) adverse events (Table 4.2).

Clinician-reported Eczema Signs

Clinician-assessed signs tend to focus on assessment of disease severity. More than 20 instruments have been used to evaluate the severity of atopic dermatitis,[32] with the SCORing Atopic Dermatitis Index (SCORAD),[13] Eczema Area Severity Index (EASI),[12] Investigator's Global Assessment (IGA) and Six Area, Six Sign Atopic Dermatitis (SASSAD)[14] among the most frequently used outcomes in RCTs from 1985 to 2010. The SCORAD assesses three components: (1) extent of disease; (2) severity of erythema, oedema or papulation, oozing/crusts, excoriation and lichenification and (3) subjective symptoms of pruritus and sleep loss. The SCORAD can be modified to provide an objective measure (oSCORAD) by removing assessment of subjective symptoms. Scores for each of the three domains can be summed to provide a total score.

The EASI assesses disease severity at four body sites, and measures extent of the clinical signs of erythema, induration/population, excoriation and lichenification. The IGA provides a global assessment of disease severity; however, a review of the use of IGA in atopic dermatitis clinical trials found considerable variation in nomenclature and scoring.[31] The review found the six-point scale of disease severity to be the most frequently used, with the score ranging from zero (clear) to five (very severe). The SASSAD uses a four-point scale to grade signs at six body sites: head and neck, trunk, legs, feet, arms and hands. Signs assessed are scored from zero to three for erythema, exudation, cracking, dryness, excoriation and lichenification.

The Three-item Severity scale (TIS) was designed as a short scale for measuring disease severity in clinical practice.[15] Scores between zero and three are allocated according to the severity of erythem, population/oedema and excoriation, based on the most representative lesion. A scoring system for grading atopic dermatitis severity proposed by Rajka and Langeland (1989)[16] assesses the extent, clinical course and intensity. Each factor is scored from one to three, with scores summed to provide an overall score. A score of three or four indicates mild disease, four-and-a-half to seven and a half indicates moderate severity, and a score of eight or nine indicates severe disease. Another outcome used to assess eczema is quantification of transepidermal water loss (TEWL). This measures the amount of water diffusion through the skin and is used as an indicator of skin barrier function.

Patient-reported Eczema Symptoms

The Patient-oriented Eczema Measure (POEM)[17] is the preferred outcome for assessing eczema symptoms, recommended in the HOME consensus.[11] The POEM uses a five-point scale (based on number of days) to assess the frequency of the symptoms of skin dryness, itching, flaking, cracking, bleeding, weeping/oozing and disturbed sleep. The Patient-oriented SCOring Atopic Dermatitis Index (PO-SCORAD)[18] allows for self-assessment of atopic dermatitis. Based on the SCORAD, the PO-SCORAD has been illustrated to facilitate self-completion. The PO-SCORAD has been shown to correlate well with the SCORAD index.[18]

Another tool for self-assessment of symptoms is the Self-administered Eczema Area and Severity Index (SA-EASI).[19] The SA-EASI can be completed by caregivers, and measures disease severity (based on body surface area) and visual analogue scale (VAS) scoring of skin redness, thickness, dryness, itchiness and number of scratches of an average lesion. Scores are calculated according to the patient's age and acute/chronic manifestations of lesions. The score for itching is not included in the total score.[33]

The Atopic Dermatitis Quickscore (ADQ)[20] assesses severity of skin lesions on the head, neck, trunk, arms, hands, legs and feet. Severity is scored on a six-point scale, and scores for each body area are added together to give a total score. A score for evaluation of pruritus severity is also allocated for the same body areas. The scores for both skin lesion and pruritus severity are added together to provide a total score.

The Nottingham Eczema Severity Score (NESS)[21] was adapted from the index developed by Rajka and Langeland,[16] and measures the extent of atopic dermatitis combined with intensity and frequency. The Itch Severity Scale (ISS)[22] measures itch frequency, duration, pattern, involved body surface area, itch intensity (using a five-point Likert scale and VAS), itch sensation, current treatments and efficacy, and impact on various aspects of life including sleep, diet, and sexual desire and function.

Long-term Control

Long-term control is an important outcome for atopic dermatitis; however, there is currently no consensus on how this should be measured.[11] Approaches adopted in clinical studies include evaluating the rate of relapse and monitoring the time to recurrence of symptoms.

Health-related Quality of Life

The physical and psychological burden from atopic dermatitis is considerable. While assessment of health-related quality of life (HRQoL) is important, no consensus on which instrument should be used has been reached.[11] One outcome tool that assesses HRQoL specific to atopic dermatitis is the Quality of Life Index for Atopic Dermatitis (QoLIAD).[23] The QoLIAD is a 25-item questionnaire which measures the impact of functional impairment on quality of life.

Several other HRQoL tools can be used for dermatology. The Dermatology Life Quality Index (DLQI)[25] uses a four-point scale to assess the impact of atopic dermatitis on symptoms and feelings, daily activities, leisure, school or work, personal relationships and the impact of treatment. The DLQI was adapted for use in children (the Children's Dermatology Life Quality Index, CDLQI).[26] The

CDLQI also uses a four-point scale, but questions related to adult activities like shopping or looking after the home were replaced with questions about friendships, teasing/bullying and sleep. Versions of the Skindex[24] include the 29- and 16-item versions. Scores are allocated in domains for symptoms, emotions and function. The domain and total scores can be converted to a linear scale of zero to 100.

Two commonly used generic well-being questionnaires are the Medical Outcome Study Short Form 36-item questionnaire (SF-36)[27] and the EuroQoL-5 Dimensions questionnaire (EQ-5D).[28] The SF-36 includes 36 items relating to eight domains: (1) physical functioning; (2) role functioning due to health problems; (3) role functioning due to emotional problems; (4) bodily pain; (5) general health perceptions; (6) vitality; (7) social function; and (8) mental health. The EQ-5D includes five questions related to mobility, self-care, usual activities, pain or discomfort, and anxiety or depression. The EQ-5D also includes a 100-point VAS to assess overall health status. Results can be presented in a variety of ways. For the five domains, a higher score indicates a greater level of perceived problems, while for the VAS component, a higher score indicates better health status.

Effective Rate

Effective rate is an outcome which provides an overall assessment of symptom change. Two guidelines were selected for inclusion: *Criteria of Diagnosis and Therapeutic Effect of Diseases and Syndromes in Traditional Chinese Medicine* 中医病证诊断疗效标准 (1994 guideline)[29] and the *Guideline for Clinical Research of Traditional Chinese Medicine New Drugs* 中药新药临床研究指导原则(试行) (2002 guideline).[30] The 1994 guideline describes three categories for determining clinical effect:

- Cure: Skin rash subsided, residual pigmentation or plaque.
- Improved: Skin lesions thinning, faded in color, subsided by more than 30%, and itching reduced.
- Not improved: Skin lesions subsided less than 30%.

To determine the effective rate, the number of people achieving 'cure' and 'improved' are summed up.

The 2002 guideline describes three approaches for determining the effective rate. The first approach uses a formula to calculate overall therapeutic effectiveness for the disease. The calculation method is (pre-treatment scores — post-treatment scores)/pre-treatment scores X 100%. The score used in this calculation is an overall assessment of four factors: itch severity, rash distribution, acute/chronic phase and laboratory examinations. The criteria used to determine therapeutic efficiency are as follows:

- Clinical cure: All the skin lesions have disappeared, symptoms have disappeared, laboratory testing returned to normal and total scores decreased more than 95%.
- Remarkable effect: Most of the skin lesions have subsided, symptoms have improved significantly or laboratory testing nearly returned to normal, and total scores decreased more than 70% and less than 95%.
- Effective: Part of the skin lesions have subsided, symptoms partly improved and total scores decreased more than 50% and less than 70%.
- Invalid: Skin lesion improvement is not obvious, symptoms are not improved, or may have worsened, and the total scores decreased less than 50%.

To determine the effective rate, the numbers of people achieving 'clinical cure,' 'remarkable effect' and "effective" are summed up.

The second approach evaluates two individual symptoms: itch and skin lesion area. The criteria for assessing change in itch are as follows:

- Recovery: No itch.
- Remarkable effect: The pruritic grade decreased by two levels.
- Effective: The pruritic grade decreased by one level.
- Invalid: The pruritic grade did not decrease, or may have worsened.

The criteria for assessing change in lesion area are as follows:

- Recovery: Completely restored normal skin or some pigmentation exists.
- Remarkable effect: Skin lesion area reduced more than 70% but less than 100%.
- Effective: Skin lesion area reduced more than 50% but less than 70%.
- Invalid: Skin lesion area reduced less than 50% or may have expanded.

To determine the effective rate, the numbers of people achieving 'recovery,' 'remarkable effect,' and "effective" are summed up.

The third approach relates to change in CM syndrome. As this is more challenging to evaluate and interpret clinically, data using this approach were not extracted.

Adverse Events

Adverse events are an important outcome for skin conditions such as atopic dermatitis, as some pharmacological treatments have been associated with increased adverse events. Information about the nature and number of adverse events was included where noted.

Risk of Bias Assessment

Risk of bias was assessed for RCTs using the Cochrane Collaboration's tool.[1] In clinical trials, bias can be categorised as selection bias, performance bias, detection bias, attrition bias and reporting bias. Each domain is assessed to determine whether the bias is at 'low,' 'high' or 'unclear' risk. 'Low' risk of bias indicates that bias is unlikely, 'high' risk indicates plausible bias that seriously weakens confidence in the results and 'unclear' bias indicates lack of information or uncertainty over potential bias and raises some doubt about the results. Risk of bias assessment was verified by two people and disagreement was resolved by discussion or consultation with a third person.

Risk of bias is categorised using the following six domains:

- Sequence generation: The method used to generate the allocation sequence is given in sufficient detail to allow an assessment of whether it should produce comparable groups. 'Low' risk of bias refers to a random number table or computer random generator. 'High' risk of bias includes studies that describe a non-random sequence generation, such as odd or even date of birth or date of admission.
- Allocation concealment: The method used to conceal the allocation sequence is given in enough detail to determine whether intervention allocations could have been foreseen before or during enrolment. 'Low' risk of bias includes central randomisation or sealed envelopes and 'high' risk of bias includes open random sequence, etc.
- Blinding of participants and personnel: Measures used to describe if the study participants and personnel are blind to the intervention received. In addition, information relating to whether the blinding was effective is also assessed. Studies that ensure blinding of participants and personnel are at 'low' risk of bias. If the study is not blind, or incompletely blind, it is at 'high' risk of bias.
- Blinding of outcome assessors: Measures used to describe if the outcome assessors are blind to knowledge of which intervention a participant received. In addition, information relating to whether the blinding was effective is also assessed. Studies that ensure blinding of outcome assessors are at 'low' risk of bias. If the study is not blind, or incompletely blind, it is at 'high' risk of bias.
- Incomplete outcome data: Completeness of outcome data for each main outcome including drop outs, exclusions from the analysis with numbers missing in each group and reasons for drop out or exclusions. Studies with 'low' risk of bias would include all outcome data, or if there is missing data it is unlikely to relate to the true outcome or is balanced between groups. Studies at 'high' risk of bias would have unexplained missing data.
- Selective reporting: The study protocol is available and the pre-specified outcomes are included in the report. Studies with a

published protocol, and which include all pre-specified outcomes in their report, would be at 'low' risk of bias. Studies at 'high' risk of bias would not include all pre-specified outcomes or the outcome data may be reported incompletely.

Statistical Analyses

Frequency of CM syndromes, CHM formulas, herbs and acupuncture points reported in included studies are presented using descriptive statistics. Chinese medicine syndromes reported in two or more studies were presented. The ten most frequently reported CHM formulas and 20 most frequently reported herbs presented were used in at least two studies, although for CHM formulas this was not always possible. The top ten acupuncture points used in two or more studies are presented, or as available. Where data was limited, reports of single CM syndromes or acupuncture points were provided as a guide for the reader.

Definitions of statistical tests and results are described in the glossary. Dichotomous data are reported as a risk ratio (RR) with 95% confidence interval (CI), and continuous data are reported as mean difference (MD), or standardised mean difference (SMD), with 95% CI. For dichotomous data, when the RR is greater than one and the upper and lower values of the 95% CI are both greater than one, this indicates we can be 95% certain that there is a difference between the groups and that the true effect lies within these CIs. The same is true for values less than one. In such cases, we say there is a 'significant difference' between the groups. For continuous data, when the MD is greater than zero and both the upper and lower values of the 95% CI are greater than zero, we say there is a 'significant difference' between the groups. The same is true on the negative side of the scale.[1] For all analyses, RR or MD and 95% CI were reported, together with a formal test for heterogeneity using the I^2 statistic. An I^2 score greater than 50% was considered to indicate substantial heterogeneity.[1] Sensitivity analyses were undertaken to explore potential sources of heterogeneity, based on 'low' risk of bias for one of the risk of bias domains, sequence generation. Where possible and appropriate, planned subgroup analyses included duration of treatment, CM syndromes, CM formula and comparator type. Available case analysis with a random effects model was used in all analyses. The random effects model was used to take into account the clinical heterogeneity likely to be encountered within, and between, included studies, and the variation in treatment effects between included studies.

Assessment Using GRADE

The Grading of Recommendations Assessment, Development and Evaluation (GRADE) approach was used.[34] The GRADE approach summarises and rates the strength and quality of evidence ('certainty') in systematic reviews using a structured process for presenting evidence summaries. The results are presented in summary of findings tables. The results provide an important overview for atopic dermatitis outcomes.

A panel of experts was established to evaluate the strength and quality of evidence. The panel included the systematic review team, CM practitioners, integrative medicine experts, research methodologists and conventional medicine physicians. The experts were asked to rate the clinical importance of key interventions from CHM, acupuncture therapies and other CM therapies, as well as comparators and outcomes. Results were collated and, based on the rating scores and subsequent discussion, a consensus on the content for the summary of findings tables was achieved.

The certainty of evidence for each outcome was rated according to five factors outlined in the GRADE approach. The certainty of evidence may be rated based on:

- Limitations in study design (risk of bias).
- Inconsistency of results (unexplained heterogeneity).
- Indirectness of evidence (interventions, populations and outcomes important to the patients with the condition).
- Imprecision (uncertainty about the results).
- Publication bias (selective publication of studies).

These five factors are additive, and a reduction in more than one factor will reduce the certainty of the evidence for that outcome. The

GRADE approach also includes three domains that can be rated up, including large magnitude of an effect, dose-response gradient and effect of plausible residual confounding. However, these three domains relate to observational studies including cohort, case-control, before-after and time-series studies. The GRADE summaries in this book include only RCTs; therefore, these three domains for rating up were not assessed.

Treatment recommendations can also be assessed using the GRADE approach; however, due to the diverse nature of CM practice, treatment recommendations were not included with the summary of findings. Therefore, the reader should interpret the evidence with reference to the local practice environment. It should also be noted that the GRADE approach requires judgments about the certainty of evidence and some subjective assessment. However, the experience of the panel members suggests the judgments are reliable and are transparent representations of the certainty of evidence.

The GRADE levels of evidence are grouped into four categories:

1. 'High' certainty: We are very confident that the true effect lies close to that of the estimate of the effect.
2. 'Moderate' certainty: We are moderately confident in the effect estimate; the true effect is likely to be close to the estimate of the effect, but there is a possibility that it is substantially different.
3. 'Low' certainty: Our confidence in the effect estimate is limited; the true effect may be substantially different from the estimate of the effect.
4. 'Very low' certainty: We have very little confidence in the effect estimate; the true effect is likely to be substantially different from the estimate of effect.

References

1. Higgins JPT, Green S, eds. (2011) Cochrane Handbook for Systematic Reviews of Interventions Version 5.1.0 [updated March 2011]. The Cochrane Collaboration. Available from: www.cochrane-handbook. org2011.

2. Williams HC, Burney PG, Hay RJ, *et al.* (1994) The UK Working Party's Diagnostic Criteria for Atopic Dermatitis. I. Derivation of a minimum set of discriminators for atopic dermatitis. *Br J Dermatol* **131**(3): 383–396.

3. Hanifin J, Rajka G. (1980) Diagnostic features of atopic eczema. *Acta Dermatol Venereol* **92**: 44–47.

4. Eichenfield LF, Tom WL, Berger TG, *et al.* (2014) Guidelines of care for the management of atopic dermatitis: Section 2. Management and treatment of atopic dermatitis with topical therapies. *J Am Acad Dermatol* **71**(1): 116–132.

5. Sidbury R, Davis DM, Cohen DE, *et al.* (2014) Guidelines of care for the management of atopic dermatitis: Section 3. Management and treatment with phototherapy and systemic agents. *J Am Acad Dermatol* **71**(2): 327–349.

6. Sidbury R, Tom WL, Bergman JN, *et al.* (2014) Guidelines of care for the management of atopic dermatitis: Section 4. Prevention of disease flares and use of adjunctive therapies and approaches. *J Am Acad Dermatol* **71**(6): 1218–1233.

7. Katayama I, Kohno Y, Akiyama K, *et al.* (2014) Japanese guideline for atopic dermatitis 2014. *Allergol Int* **63**(3): 377–398.

8. Rubel D, Thirumoorthy T, Soebaryo RW, *et al.* (2013) Consensus guidelines for the management of atopic dermatitis: An Asia-Pacific perspective. *J Dermatol* **40**(3): 160–171.

9. Saeki H, Nakahara T, Tanaka A, *et al.* (2016) Clinical practice guidelines for the management of atopic dermatitis 2016. *J Dermatol* **43**(10): 1117–1145.

10. Werfel T, Heratizadeh A, Aberer W, *et al.* (2016) S2k guideline on diagnosis and treatment of atopic dermatitis: Short version. *J Dtsch Dermatol Ges* **14**(1): 92–106.

11. Chalmers JR, Simpson E, Apfelbacher CJ, *et al.* (2016) Report from the fourth international consensus meeting to harmonize core outcome measures for atopic eczema/dermatitis clinical trials (HOME initiative). *Br J Dermatol* **175**(1): 69–79.

12. Tofte S, Graeber M, Cherill R, *et al.* (1998) Eczema area and severity index (EASI): A new tool to evaluate atopic dermatitis. *J Eur Acad Dermatol Venereol* **11**: S197.

13. (1993) Severity scoring of atopic dermatitis: The SCORAD index. Consensus Report of the European Task Force on Atopic Dermatitis. *Dermatology* **186**: 23–31.

14. Berth-Jones J. (1996) Six area, six sign atopic dermatitis (SASSAD) severity score: A simple system for monitoring disease activity in atopic dermatitis. *Br J Dermatol* **135**(Suppl 48): 25–30.
15. Wolkerstorfer A, de Waard Van der Spek FB, Glazenburg EJ, *et al.* (1999) Scoring the severity of atopic dermatitis: Three item severity score as a rough system for daily practice and as a pre-screening tool for studies. *Acta Dermatol Venereol* **79**(5): 356–359.
16. Rajka G, Langeland T. (1989) Grading of the severity of atopic dermatitis. *Acta Dermatol Venereol Suppl (Stockholm)* **144**: 13–14.
17. Charman CR, Venn AJ, Williams HC. (2004) The patient-oriented eczema measure: Development and initial validation of a new tool for measuring atopic eczema severity from the patients' perspective. *Arch Dermatol* **140**(12): 1513–1519.
18. Stalder JF, Barbarot S, Wollenberg A, *et al.* (2011) Patient-Oriented SCORAD (PO-SCORAD): A new self-assessment scale in atopic dermatitis validated in Europe. *Allergy* **66**(8): 1114–1121.
19. Housman TS, Patel MJ, Camacho F, *et al.* (2002) Use of the Self-Administered Eczema Area and Severity Index by parent caregivers: Results of a validation study. *Br J Dermatol* **147**(6): 1192–1198.
20. Carel K, Bratton DL, Miyazawa N, *et al.* (2008) The Atopic Dermatitis Quickscore (ADQ): Validation of a new parent-administered atopic dermatitis scoring tool. *Ann Allergy Asthma Immunol* **101**(5): 500–507.
21. Emerson RM, Charman CR, Williams HC. (2000) The Nottingham Eczema Severity Score: Preliminary refinement of the Rajka and Langeland grading. *Br J Dermatol* **142**(2): 288–297.
22. Majeski CJ, Johnson JA, Davison SN, *et al.* (2007) Itch Severity Scale: A self-report instrument for the measurement of pruritus severity. *Br J Dermatol* **156**(4): 667–673.
23. Whalley D, McKenna SP, Dewar AL, *et al.* (2004) A new instrument for assessing quality of life in atopic dermatitis: International development of the Quality of Life Index for Atopic Dermatitis (QoLIAD). *Br J Dermatol* **150**(2): 274–283.
24. Chren MM, Lasek RJ, Quinn LM, *et al.* (1996) Skindex, a quality-of-life measure for patients with skin disease: Reliability, validity, and responsiveness. *J Invest Dermatol* **107**(5): 707–713.
25. Finlay A, Khan G. (1994) Dermatology Life Quality Index (DLQI): A simple practical measure for routine clinical use. *Clin Exp Dermatol* **19**(3): 210–216.

26. Lewis-Jones MS, Finlay AY. (1995) The Children's Dermatology Life Quality Index (CDLQI): Initial validation and practical use. *Br J Dermatol* **132**(6): 942–949.

27. Ware JJ, Sherbourne C. (1992) The MOS 36-item short-form health survey (SF-36). I. Conceptual framework and item selection. *Med Care* **30**: 473–483.

28. Rabin R, de Charro F. (2001) EQ-5D: A measure of health status from the EuroQol Group. *Ann Med* **33**: 337–343.

29. 国家中医药管理局. (1994) 中医病证诊断疗效标准. 南京 : 南京大学出版社.

30. 郑筱萸. (2002) 中药新药临床研究指导原则（试行). 北京 : 中国医药科技出版社.

31. Futamura M, Leshem YA, Thomas KS, *et al.* (2016) A systematic review of Investigator Global Assessment (IGA) in atopic dermatitis (AD) trials: Many options, no standards. *J Am Acad Dermatol* **74**(2): 288–294.

32. Rehal B, Armstrong AW. (2012) Health outcomes in atopic dermatitis. *Dermatol Clin* **30**(1): 73–86, viii.

33. Van Velsen SG, Knol MJ, Haeck IM, *et al.* (2010) The Self-administered Eczema Area and Severity Index in children with moderate to severe atopic dermatitis: Better estimation of AD body surface area than severity. *Pediatr Dermatol* **27**(5): 470–475.

34. Schunemann H, Brozek J, Guyatt G, Oxman A, eds. (2013) *GRADE Handbook for Grading Quality of Evidence and Strength of Recommendations*. The GRADE Working Group. Available from: http://www.guidelinedevelopment.org/handbook/.

5

Clinical Evidence for Chinese Herbal Medicine

OVERVIEW

The body of literature for the treatment of atopic dermatitis using Chinese herbal medicine is growing. Many clinical studies have evaluated Chinese herbal medicine, and this chapter reviews the treatments, efficacy and safety from 162 studies published in scientific journals. The majority of studies have evaluated oral Chinese herbal medicine, which has shown promising results in reducing the signs and symptoms of atopic dermatitis.

Introduction

Chinese herbal medicine (CHM) was commonly used in classical literature (see Chapter 3) and continues to be used to treat skin conditions including atopic dermatitis. In recent years many clinical studies have been conducted that have examined the potential benefit of CHM. These have been published in Chinese and international scientific journals. Reviews of the clinical evidence have been grouped according to the route of administration. Studies of oral CHM are presented first, followed by topical CHM, and concluding with the combination of oral plus topical CHM.

Previous Systematic Reviews

Many systematic reviews (SRs) have evaluated the efficacy of CHM for atopic eczema. Five SRs were identified from the English literature,[1–5] and three SRs were found through the Chinese databases.[6-8] Reviews published in English have highlighted the low methodological quality of included studies as a factor limiting the certainty of findings.[2-5] The most recent review of 24 randomised controlled trials (RCTs) by Shi *et al.* (2017)[4] included studies of CHM, acupuncture and other Chinese medicine (CM) therapies. Meta-analyses included different types of interventions, and no evidence was presented specifically for CHM.

Ten RCTs were included in the review of topical CHM by Gu *et al.* (2014).[3] The rate of adverse events was lower with CHM, compared with the control groups. While some benefit was seen with topical CHM in improving the total effective rate, the authors concluded that methodological weakness of the included studies limited the certainty of the findings. A similar finding was reached in a Cochrane review of 28 RCTs of CHM for atopic eczema.[2] Chinese herbal medicine showed some benefit in improving clinical effect and itch compared with placebo or conventional medicines. No difference was seen in the rate of adverse events in two studies. The low to very low quality of included studies limited the reliability of the results, leading the authors to state there was no conclusive evidence that CHM improved eczema severity.

Tan *et al.* (2013)[5] reviewed the efficacy and safety of CHM for atopic dermatitis in seven RCTs. Compared with placebo, CHM reduced the severity of erythema and surface damage in three studies, reduced pruritus in one study, improved sleep score in one study and improved quality of life on the Children's Dermatology Life Quality Index (CDLQI) in one study. No adverse events were reported in the included studies. The review highlighted that studies addressing methodological issues are needed. An earlier review of two RCTs was conducted by Armstrong and Ernst (1999).[1] Both RCTs showed benefit for atopic dermatitis with CHM; however, data were not subject to meta-analysis.

Three reviews published in Chinese evaluated oral[6,7] and topical CHM.[8] Thirteen RCTs were included in the review of oral CHM by Yang *et al.* (2016).[6] The review found greater improvement in patients' symptoms with CHM compared to conventional medicine. In addition, the effective rate was higher with CHM and fewer adverse reactions were seen with CHM than conventional medicine. The authors concluded that methodological weakness of the included studies limited the certainty of the findings. Similar findings were seen in a review by Gong *et al.* (2009).[7] Eleven RCTs were included, and the results showed the efficacy of CHM was greater than antihistamines. Sensitivity analysis determined the conclusions of the study to be credible.

Fourteen RCTs were included in the review of topical CHM by Wu *et al.* (2015).[8] The effective rate with CHM was better than that of the control groups, which included treatment with various pharmacotherapies. The adverse event rate in eight studies and recurrence rate in three studies were lower with topical CHM than in the control groups. The review highlighted methodological issues in the included RCTs.

Identification of Clinical Studies

A comprehensive search of nine electronic databases and four clinical trial registries identified 17,364 potentially relevant citations. After duplicates were removed, a further 7,600 citations were excluded after reviewing the title and abstract. The full text of 539 articles was read to assess study eligibility. In total, 166 studies met the inclusion criteria for this chapter. Ninety-three of these were RCTs, 11 were non-randomised controlled clinical trials (CCTs) and 62 were non-controlled studies. Four studies (two RCTs and two non-controlled studies) were identified using CHM interventions not commonly practised outside of China and were excluded from subsequent analysis. The findings of 162 studies are described in this chapter. The process for selection of studies is shown in Fig. 5.1. Included studies are referred to in the text by an 'H' followed by a number, for example 'H1.' The reference list for included studies can be found at the end of this chapter.

Oral Chinese Herbal Medicine

Oral CHM was the most frequently evaluated route of administration, used in 91 of the included studies. These studies included 6,564 participants. Oral CHM was administered in 51 of the included RCTs (H1–H51), in six CCTs (H52–H57), and 36 non-controlled studies (H58–H93).

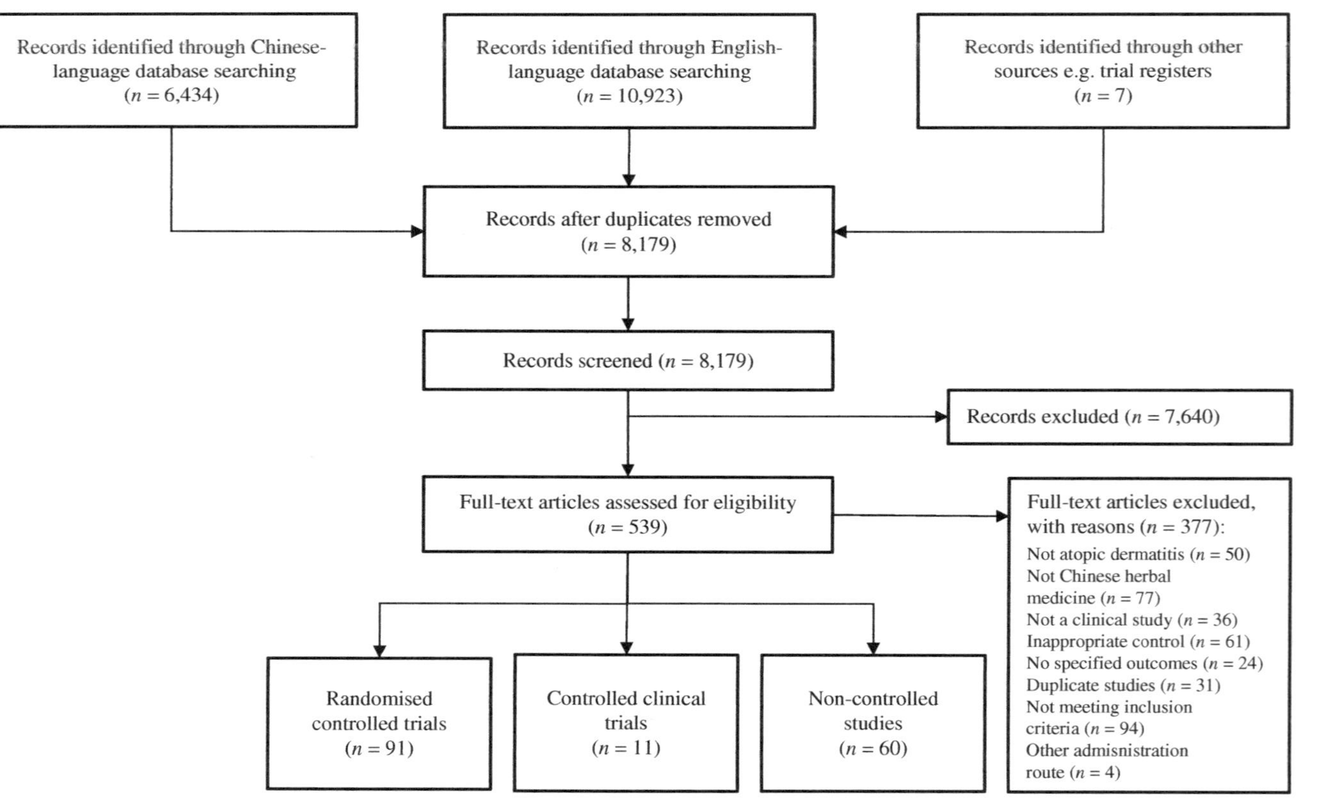

Fig. 5.1. Flowchart of study selection process: Chinese herbal medicine.

Randomised Controlled Trials of Oral Chinese Herbal Medicine

In total, 5,073 people participated in the 51 RCTs of oral CHM (H1–H51). Forty-eight RCTs used a two-arm parallel group design. Two studies (H20, H51) included two treatment arms (three arms in total), with one arm receiving oral CHM and the other receiving oral plus topical CHM. Information for the oral CHM arm is presented here, with details for the oral plus topical CHM included below. Another study (H30) included four arms: two treatment arms of oral CHM alone and oral CHM as an integrative medicine (IM, where CHM is used in combination with at least one guideline-recommended treatment), and two comparator arms of narrow band ultra-violet B (NB-UVB) and the antihistamine loratadine. In analysis of the results, comparisons were made for CHM vs. NB-UVB, CHM as an IM vs. NB-UVB, and CHM vs. loratadine.

The majority of the studies were conducted in mainland China, with two studies (H48, H49) conducted in Hong Kong, two studies (H14, H47) in Taiwan and one study (H50) in Japan. The majority of studies were conducted in outpatient departments, with one study (H13) recruiting participants from the inpatient department and three studies (H21, H30, H43) recruiting participants from both inpatient and outpatient departments. The time living with atopic dermatitis varied across studies from one week (H3) to 40 years (H17, H45). Participant age ranged from six months (H3) to 70 years (H2) in studies that reported this information, with a median age of 13.4 years. In studies that reported participant gender, there were more males than females (1,922 males compared to 1,620 females).

Duration of treatment with oral CHM varied across studies, ranging from 14 days (H3) to 24 weeks (H50). The majority of studies administered oral CHM for one month or less (31 studies: H1, H2, H6–H12, H14–H16, H18, H19, H22–H25, H27–H29, H31, H32, H37, H39–H45). Follow-up assessment was conducted in 21 studies (H3, H6, H7, H9–H12, H14, H17, H19–H21, H25, H28, H29, H38, H42, H43, H47, H49, H51), and ranged from four weeks (H47) to one year (H6) after the end of treatment. Ten studies (H3, H7, H12,

H40, H41, H47–H51) reported loss to follow-up, with all but two studies (H47, H51) reporting rates of attrition less than 10%. Both studies reported reasons for participant withdrawal, which included compliance issues, being unable/unwilling to continue the study, family reasons and receiving/not receiving benefit from the treatment.

Chinese medicine syndrome differentiation was used as an inclusion criterion in 17 studies (H1, H3, H4, H7, H14, H15, H19, H21, H23–H25, H28, H34, H36, H38, H41, H43), with all studies only describing one syndrome. Two syndromes were described in four studies: Spleen deficiency syndrome (H7, H19, H25, H43) and Spleen deficiency with dampness accumulation/retention/stagnation (H1, H3, H4, H15). Other syndromes included Spleen deficiency with Blood dryness (H23, H24, H36), wind-damp-heat (H14, H21), Blood deficiency with wind-dryness (H34, H38), Spleen deficiency with damp-heat (H28) and *yin* injury syndrome (H41). Fewer studies described using syndrome differentiation to guide treatment, although all described multiple syndromes. Blood deficiency and wind-dryness were described in three studies (H16, H32, H37), as was damp-heat accumulation/encumbrance (H32, H37). Other syndromes reported in one study included Spleen deficiency with dampness retention (H16), Spleen dampness (H39), damp-heat accumulation due to dysfunction of the Spleen in transportation (H12), Lung deficiency with skin dryness and wind-heat with damp (H12), wind-heat with damp (H16), Spleen deficiency (H32), foetal heat syndrome (heat transferred from the mother *in utero*, H39), *yin* deficiency and Blood dryness (H39), relative predominance of Heart fire (H51) and relative predominance of Spleen deficiency (H51).

Oral CHM was used alone in 25 studies (H3, H5, H8–H10, H13–H15, H17, H19, H20, H22, H24, H27, H30, H34, H36–H38, H41, H47–H51), and as an IM in 27 studies (H1, H2, H4, H6, H7, H11, H12, H16, H18, H21, H23, H25, H26, H28–H33, H35, H39, H40, H42–H46). One study (H30) evaluated oral CHM alone and as an IM. Many of the studies evaluated CHM formulas that were developed by study investigators. Unnamed formulas were excluded from formula frequency analysis. Forty-one different formulas were evaluated, with several being tested in multiple studies. One commercial product, compound glycyrrhizin 复方甘草酸苷片 was evaluated in four studies

(H2, H29, H31, H42) (Table 5.1). Other formulas tested in multiple studies included *Xiao feng san* 消风散, *Dang gui yin zi* 当归饮子, *Si wu tang* 四物汤加减, *Long dan xie gan tang* 龙胆泻肝汤加减 and *Jian pi hua shi tang* 健脾化湿汤 (an investigator-developed formula).

Table 5.1.   Frequently Reported Oral Formulas in Randomised Controlled Trials

Most Common Formulas/Products	No. of Studies	Ingredients
Fu fang gan cao suan gan pian 复方甘草酸苷片	4	Compound glycyrrhizin 甘草酸苷 (H2, H29, H31, H42)
Xiao feng san 消风散	4	*Dang gui* 当归, *sheng di huang* 生地黄, *fang feng* 防风, *chan tui* 蝉蜕, *zhi mu* 知母, *ku shen* 苦参, *hu ma* 胡麻, *jing jie* 荆芥, *cang zhu* 苍朮, *niu bang zi* 牛蒡子, *shi gao* 石膏, *gan cao* 甘草 and *mu tong* 木通
Dang gui yin zi 当归饮子	3	*Dang gui* 当归, *bai shao* 白芍, *chuan xiong* 川芎, *sheng di huang* 生地黄, *bai ji li* 白蒺藜, *fang feng* 防风, *jing jie* 荆芥, *huang qi* 黄芪, *he shou wu* 何首乌 and *gan cao* 甘草
Si wu tang (modified) 四物汤加减	2	*Bai shao* 白芍, *dang gui* 当归, *shu di huang* 熟地黄 and *chuan xiong* 川芎
Long dan xie gan tang 龙胆泻肝汤加减	2	*Long dan cao* 龙胆草, *zhi zi* 栀子, *huang qin* 黄芩, *mu tong* 木通, *ze xie* 泽泻, *che qian zi* 车前子, *sheng di* 生地, *dang gui* 当归, *gan cao* 甘草 and *chai hu* 柴胡
Jian pi hua shi tang 健脾化湿汤	2	*Tai zi shen* 太子参, *chao bai zhu* 炒白术, *fu ling* 茯苓, *chao yi yi ren* 炒薏苡仁, *chen pi* 陈皮, *cang zhu* 苍术, *bai ji li* 白蒺藜, *fang feng* 防风, *bai xian pi* 白鲜皮, *dan zhu ye* 淡竹叶 and *sheng mu li* 生牡蛎 (H4, H33)

Note: (1) The use of the some herbs may be restricted in some countries. Readers are advised to comply with relevant regulations and (2) Studies using these formulas varied in the listed herb ingredients. Ingredients listed in Table 5.1 are sourced from original studies where available, and the study reference noted in brackets. Where ingredients were not available, or where the ingredients differed among studies describing the same formula name, herb ingredients were sourced from the *Zhong Yi Fang Ji Da Ci Dian* 中医方剂大辞典.

One hundred and five different herbs were used in the 51 RCTs. The most frequently used herb was *gan cao* 甘草, including related herbs such as *gan cao suan gan* 甘草酸苷 (Table 5.2). In addition to *gan cao* 甘草, other herbs used frequently in oral CHM RCTs included *bai zhu* 白术, *fu ling* 茯苓, *dang gui* 当归, and *yi yi ren* 薏苡仁.

Table 5.2. Frequently Reported Orally Used Herbs in Randomised Controlled Trials

Most Common Herbs	Scientific Name	Frequency of Use
Gan cao 甘草	*Glycyrrhiza* spp	37
Bai zhu 白术	*Atractylodes macrocephala* Koidz.	28
Fu ling 茯苓	*Poria cocos* (Schw.) Wolf	28
Dang gui 当归	*Angelica sinensis* (Oliv.) Diels	26
Yi yi ren 薏苡仁	*Coix lacryma-jobi* L. var. mayuen (Roman.) Stapf	25
Sheng di huang 生地黄	*Rehmannia glutinosa* Libosch.	24
Fang feng 防风	*Saposhnikovia divaricata* (Turcz.) Schischk.	24
Bai xian pi 白鲜皮	*Dictamnus dasycarpus* Turcz.	23
Cang zhu 苍术	*Atractylodes* spp	20
Huang qi 黄芪	*Astragalus* spp	18
Jing jie 荆芥	*Schizonepeta tenuifolia* Briq.	16
Ci ji li 刺蒺藜 (*bai ji li* 白蒺藜)	*Tribulus terrestris* L.	15 (10)
Ku shen 苦参	*Sophora flavescens* Ait.	15
Huang qin 黄芩	*Scutellaria baicalensis* Georgi	15
Ze xie 泽泻	*Alisma orientalis* (Sam.) Juzep.	13
Chan tui 蝉蜕	*Cryptotympana pustulata* Fabricius	13
Di fu zi 地肤子	*Kochia scoparia* (L.) Schrad.	11
Dan shen 丹参	*Salvia miltiorrhiza* Bge.	9
Bai shao 白芍	*Paeonia lactiflora* Pall.	9

Note: The use of some herbs may be restricted in some countries. Readers are advised to comply with relevant regulations.

In all studies, the treatment delivered in the comparator group included at least one guideline recommended treatment (including emollients) or placebo. Pharmacotherapy included topical corticosteroids (TCS) and antihistamines. Some studies also combined guideline-recommended treatments with other agents, such as vitamin B1 (H45) or C (H9, H27, H32, H37, H45), and urea ointment (H32). Three studies used light therapy in the comparator arm. Two studies (H26, H30) compared oral CHM with NB-UVB and one (H21) combined laser therapy with other pharmacotherapy. Four studies (H47–H50) compared oral CHM with placebo and three (H20, H25, H51) used both placebo and pharmacotherapy as the comparator.

Risk of Bias

All studies were described as using 'random' allocation. Fourteen studies were judged as low risk of bias for sequence generation as they used appropriate methods to allocate participants to groups (Table 5.3). These included a random number table (H3, H4, H6, H13, H18, H23, H35, H36, H38, H40, H42) or computer randomisation (H47, H49, H51). Three studies appropriately concealed group allocation through using central randomisation (H49, H51) or sealed envelopes (H47), and were judged as low risk of bias. Five studies (H25, H47–H50) used methods to blind participants to group allocation, posing low risk of bias. All remaining studies were judged as high risk due to lack of blinding of participants (H20, H21, H51), high likelihood that the blinding could be broken in studies described as single due to the nature of the interventions, and comparators preventing blinding (H1–H24, H26–H46, H51).

Four studies (H25, H49–H51) blinded research personnel to group allocation and were judged to pose low risk of bias. Two studies (H47, H48) provided insufficient detail to make an assessment and were judged as unclear risk. Two studies (H20, H21) were judged high risk as they did not blind personnel to group allocation, and the remaining studies were judged high risk due to the nature of the treatments. Six studies (low risk: H4, H25, H47–H49, H51)

Table 5.3. Risk of Bias of Randomised Controlled Trials: Oral Chinese Herbal Medicine

Risk of Bias Domain	Low Risk n (%)	Unclear Risk n (%)	High Risk n (%)
Sequence generation	14 (27.5)	37 (72.5)	0 (0)
Allocation concealment	3 (5.9)	48 (94.1)	0 (0)
Blinding of participants	5 (9.8)	0 (0)	46 (90.2)
Blinding of personnel	4 (7.8)	2 (3.9)	45 (88.2)
Blinding of outcome assessors	6 (11.8)	43 (84.3)	2 (3.9)
Incomplete outcome data	47 (92.2)	2 (3.9)	2 (3.9)
Selective outcome reporting	1 (2.0)	48 (94.1)	2 (3.9)

blinded outcome assessors to group allocation, two studies (high risk: H14, H21) did not blind outcome assessors and there was insufficient information for the remaining studies.

Most studies reported no participant loss and were judged low risk for incomplete outcome data. Two studies (H48, H50) reported loss to follow-up but did not specify which groups these participants were from, nor whether missing data were accounted for; both studies were judged as unclear risk. A further two studies were judged as high risk due to an imbalance in missing data across groups with no intention to treat analysis conducted (H3) and due to a lack of information about group allocation and reasons for withdrawal (H4). One trial (H51) was judged low risk for selective outcome reporting, as the trial was registered with the Chinese Clinical Trial Register and all specified outcomes were reported. Two studies (H28, H31) were judged as high risk as some outcomes described in the methods were not reported. For the remaining studies, no protocols were able to be identified to determine the level of risk for selective outcome reporting. In addition, two studies (H11, H28) had other sources of bias that may affect the reliability of the results. Both studies had large differences in the number of participants in each group, and neither study reported the randomisation ratio.

Outcomes

All studies reported at least one of the pre-specified outcomes. The SCORing Atopic Dermatitis Index (SCORAD)[9] was the most common outcome for assessing clinical signs, used in 16 studies. Twelve studies evaluated patient-reported symptoms, focusing on itch and sleep loss. Recurrence was evaluated in 16 studies and effective rate, using the 1994[10] and 2002[11] guidelines, was examined in 20 studies. Despite atopic dermatitis having a significant burden on health-related quality of life (HRQoL), only six studies reported this outcome. Adverse events were reported in 28 studies and are described below.

SCORing Atopic Dermatitis Index

Sixteen studies (H4, H8, H13, H19, H20, H24–H26, H30, H33–H35, H38, H41, H49, H51) reported on SCORAD.[9] Eleven of these (H8, H13, H19, H20, H24, H30, H34, H38, H41, H49, H51) evaluated oral CHM alone, and six studies (H4, H25, H26, H30, H33, H35) evaluated oral CHM as an IM. One study included two treatment arms, with one group receiving oral CHM alone and the other receiving oral CHM as an IM. Meta-analysis was conducted where possible, and results of single studies were described when not included in the meta-analysis.

Oral Chinese herbal medicine alone

Eight studies (H8, H13, H19, H24, H30, H34, H38, H41) that evaluated SCORAD compared oral CHM with guideline-recommended pharmacotherapy. Atopic dermatitis severity on SCORAD was 11.23 points lower with oral CHM than with pharmacotherapy (eight studies, 622 participants [–16.90, –5.56], $I^2 = 93\%$), although considerable statistical heterogeneity was noted (Table 5.4). This was explored through planned subgroup and sensitivity analyses. Statistical heterogeneity was reduced to moderate levels ($I^2 = 46\%$) when studies assessed as low risk of bias for sequence generation were analysed. While the number of studies

Table 5.4. Oral Chinese Herbal Medicine vs. Pharmacotherapy: SCORing Atopic Dermatitis Index

Studies	No. of Studies (Participants)	Effect Size (MD [95% CI], I^2)	Included Studies
All studies	8 (622)	−11.23 [−16.90, −5.56]*, 93%	H8, H13, H19, H24, H30, H34, H38, H41
Treatment duration: 4 wks	4 (374)	−14.02 [−20.17, −7.88]*, 81%	H8, H19, H24, H41
Treatment duration: 8 wks/2 mths	3 (184)	−8.30 [−17.45, 0.85], 93%	H30, H34, H38
Low risk of bias sequence generation	2 (120)	−13.00 [−17.64, −8.35]*, 46%	H13, H38

*Statistically significant.

Abbreviations: CI, confidence interval; MD, mean difference; mths, months; wks, weeks.

and participants was small, these may represent the most reliable evidence of the benefit of oral CHM alone for atopic dermatitis.

Two studies (H47, H49) that compared oral CHM with placebo also reported on clinical signs. An unnamed oral CHM formula was not statistically different to placebo in SCORAD score at the end of treatment (85 participants, mean difference [MD]: 2.80 points [−2.57, 8.17], H49). In the other study (H47), *Xiao feng san* 消风散 was compared with placebo in terms of clinical lesion score, erythema score and surface damage score. Results were not presented in a way that allowed for re-analysis. The study authors concluded that *Xiao feng san* 消风散 produced significant improvement in these three outcomes.

Two studies (H20, H51) compared oral CHM with placebo plus pharmacotherapy. An investigator-developed oral CHM formula produced a greater reduction in SCORAD than the combination of placebo, cetirizine and mometasone furoate (20 participants, MD: −7.62 [−11.51, −3.73], H20). The second study (H51), which compared *Pei tu qing xin tang* 培土清心汤 with placebo plus mometasone furoate, presented data in a way that did not permit re-analysis. The authors concluded that the change in SCORAD was greater in those who received *Pei tu qing xin tang* 培土清心汤 at weeks 28 and 36, than in those who received placebo plus mometasone furoate. One study (H30), with two treatment arms and two control arms, compared an investigator-developed oral CHM with NB-UVB phototherapy. In this study, the SCORAD score was lower in people who received oral CHM after treatment (61 participants, MD: –5.21 points [–9.41, –1.01]).

Oral Chinese herbal medicine as an integrative medicine

In studies that combined oral CHM with guideline-recommended pharmacotherapy, the severity of clinical signs measured using the SCORAD was 7.56 points lower with CHM than with pharmacotherapy (three studies; 275 participants, [–10.81, –4.31], $I^2 = 63\%$) (Table 5.5). Sensitivity analysis with studies assessed as low risk of bias for sequence generation was conducted to explore the substantial heterogeneity; however, statistical heterogeneity remained.

One study (H44) reported the lesion severity component of SCORAD. An investigator-developed formula as an IM resulted in a lower severity of atopic dermatitis at the end of treatment, compared with loratadine and butyric hydrocortisone (72 participants, MD: –0.52 points [–0.66, –0.38]).

Two studies (H26, H30) compared oral CHM plus NB-UVB with NB-UVB alone. The combination of oral CHM with NB-UVB produced

Table 5.5. Oral Chinese Herbal Medicine as an Integrative Medicine vs. Pharmacotherapy: SCORing Atopic Dermatitis Index

Outcomes	No. of Studies (Participants)	Effect Size (MD [95% CI], I^2)	Included Studies
All studies	3 (275)	–7.56 [–10.81, –4.31]*, 63%	H4, H33, H35
Low risk of bias sequence generation	2 (185)	–8.48 [–13.77, –3.19]*, 77%	H4, H35

*Statistically significant.
Abbreviations: CI, confidence interval; MD, mean difference.

a lower score on SCORAD at the end of treatment than NB-UVB alone (144 participants, MD: −12.24 points [−14.75, −9.73], I^2 = 0%). In one small study that compared *Jian pi shen shi* granules 健脾渗湿颗粒 as an IM with placebo and cyproheptadine, SCORAD at the end of treatment was 10.65 points lower with CHM (25 participants, [−16.24, −5.06], H25).

Eczema Area and Severity Index

Three studies (H5, H31, H43) evaluated the Eczema Area and Severity Index (EASI).[12] One study (H5) evaluated oral CHM alone, and the remaining two used oral CHM as an IM. Meta-analysis was possible for these two studies.

Oral Chinese herbal medicine alone

Modified *Xiao feng san* 消风散加减 produced a greater reduction in EASI score at the end of treatment compared to loratadine (80 participants, MD: −1.30 points [−1.48, −1.12], H5).

Oral Chinese herbal medicine as an integrative medicine

Oral CHM as an IM was not statistically different to guideline-recommended pharmacotherapy (two studies; 128 participants, MD: −1.46 points [−3.45, 0.53], I^2 = 83%, H31, H43). Substantial statistical heterogeneity was seen that was not able to be explored through subgroup analysis due to the small number of studies.

Other Measures of Clinical Signs

In addition to SCORAD and EASI, a range of other measures of clinical signs were reported. These included Six Area, Six Sign Atopic Dermatitis (SASSAD),[13] transepidermal water loss (TEWL) and scales developed by investigators. Due to the differences in measures of clinical signs, meta-analysis was not able to be conducted. Results of single studies are highlighted below.

Oral Chinese herbal medicine alone

Six studies (H3, H17, H36, H47, H48, H50) that evaluated oral CHM alone measured clinical signs. Outcome data for investigator-developed scales in the studies by Fung *et al.* (1999) (H48) and Kobayashi *et al.* (2010) (H50) were not available and were excluded from analysis. One study (H14), which measured SASSAD, used the results to calculate the effective rate of treatment, and SASSAD outcome data were not reported.

Transepidermal water loss was lower in participants who received an investigator-developed formula compared to loratadine (60 participants, MD: –9.44 g/m²h [–11.18, –7.70], H36). Using an investigator-developed scoring system, oral CHM resulted in a greater reduction in lesion area and severity, compared with loratadine (67 participants, MD: –4.11 points [–5.20, –3.02], H3). When clinical signs of itching, erythema, papules, blisters, erosions, exudation and lichenification were assessed using a four-point scale, no difference was seen between an unnamed oral CHM formula and loratadine (31 participants, MD: 0.71 points [–0.56, 1.98], H17). One study (H47) presented data in a way that did not permit re-analysis. The study authors concluded that *Xiao feng san* 消风散 was superior to placebo in reducing the total lesion score, erythema score and surface damage score.

Oral Chinese herbal medicine as an integrative medicine

Five studies (H6, H7, H21, H44, H45) that evaluated oral CHM as an IM measured clinical signs other than SCORAD and EASI. One study (H6) reported the number of people with grades zero to five (Investigator's Global Assessment) at the end of treatment. As no baseline data were available for this outcome to allow for comparison, this data were not subject to further analysis. One study (H21) used SASSAD results to determine the effective rate of treatment, but did not report the results for SASSAD. Three studies (H7, H44, H45) that compared oral CHM as an IM with pharmacotherapy used investigator-developed methods to assess clinical signs.

Itching, papules, erythema, erosion, exudation, infiltration, dryness and lichenification were assessed using a four-point scale in one RCT (H7). In 92 participants, the score for signs was 2.56 points lower in people who received *Jian pi shen shi chong ji* 健脾渗湿冲剂 as an IM compared to cyproheptadine and triamcinolone acetonide/urea ointment alone ([–3.46, –1.66]). A second study (H44) reported the lesion severity component of SCORAD. An investigator-developed formula as an IM resulted in lower atopic dermatitis severity at the end of treatment, compared with loratadine and butyric hydrocortisone (72 participants, MD: –0.52 points [–0.66, –0.38]). The third study (H45) evaluated the effect of an investigator-developed formula as an IM on erythema, papules, blisters, erosion, exudation, desquamation, scab formation and lichenification using a four-point scale. In this study, the effects of CHM as an IM were greater than those of terfenadine plus vitamins C and B1 (72 participants, MD: –1.43 points [–2.45, –0.41]).

Pruritus

Itch severity was measured using either a four-point scale (H3, H47) or on a 10-centimetre (cm) visual analogue scale (VAS) (H8, H25, H26, H34, H44). Meta-analysis was conducted using standardised mean difference (SMD) to account for differences in the way itch severity was measured.

Oral Chinese herbal medicine alone

Itch severity at the end of treatment with oral CHM was not significantly different to pharmacotherapy (three studies; 192 participants, SMD: –1.05 [–2.78, 0.67], $I^2 = 96\%$, H3, H8, H34). Due to the small number of included studies, subgroup analyses to explore potential reasons for heterogeneity were not able to be conducted. Results for itch severity in a study of *Xiao feng san* 消风散 were not able to be re-analysed (H47). The authors of this study concluded that *Xiao feng san* 消风散 produced a greater improvement in pruritus than placebo.

Oral Chinese herbal medicine as an integrative medicine

Three studies (H25, H26, H44) of oral CHM as an IM evaluated pruritus using a 10-cm VAS. Differences in comparators meant that the three studies of oral CHM as an IM were not able to be pooled for analysis. Results from single studies all showed positive results. Oral CHM, used as an IM with loratadine, resulted in an itch score 0.38 points lower than loratadine alone (72 participants, [–0.50, –0.26], H44).

One study (H25) that compared *Jian pi shen shi* granules 健脾渗湿颗粒 as an IM with placebo plus cyproheptadine reported results for itch severity on a 10-cm VAS. Itch severity at the end of treatment was 3.68 points lower with the CHM granules as an IM than with placebo plus cyproheptadine (25 participants, [–4.96, –2.40]). As an IM with NB-UVB, *ku shen* tablets 苦参片 resulted in an itch severity score at the end of treatment that was 2.00 points lower than NB-UVB alone (78 participants, [–3.12, –0.88], H26).

Sleep Disturbance

Two studies (H25, H47) reported sleep disturbance in participants with atopic dermatitis. Differences in study design meant that meta-analysis was not possible.

Oral Chinese herbal medicine alone

One study compared *Xiao feng san* 消风散 with placebo granules (H47). Sleep disturbance was rated from zero (no sleep interruptions) to four (unable to sleep) each month. Data were presented as median and interquartile range, and re-analysis was not able to be conducted. The authors reported that the improvement with *Xiao feng san* 消风散 was significantly greater than with placebo.

Oral Chinese herbal medicine as an integrative medicine

Jian pi shen shi granules 健脾渗湿颗粒 were used as an IM with cyproheptadine in one study (H25). Sleep disturbance was assessed on a 10-cm VAS, where lower scores indicated less sleep disturbance.

In this study, sleep disturbance score was 4.06 points lower at the end of treatment compared with placebo plus cyproheptadine (25 participants, [–5.76, –2.36]).

Other Patient-reported Symptoms

Five studies (H4, H33, H35, H41, H51) reported other measures of patient-reported symptoms. These included composite measures of pruritus and sleep loss, and patient self-assessment.

Oral Chinese herbal medicine alone

One study (H41) that compared an investigator-developed oral CHM formula with epinastine evaluated a composite measure of itch and sleep loss using a 10-cm VAS. In this study, oral CHM reduced the severity of itch and pruritus (60 participants, MD: –1.77 points [–3.49, –0.05]). One study (H51) that compared *Pei tu qing xin tang* 培土清心汤 with placebo plus mometasone furoate described the change in patients' self-assessment on a 10-cm VAS. The study authors concluded that the increase (improvement) in self-assessment score with *Pei tu qing xin tang* 培土清心汤 was greater than that seen with placebo plus mometasone furoate.

Oral Chinese herbal medicine as an integrative medicine

A composite measure of pruritus severity and sleep disturbance was used in three studies (H4, H33, H35). Both items were assessed on a 10-cm VAS (lower is better), and scores summed up to provide a total score. Oral CHM as an IM resulted in a lower score than pharmacotherapy alone (275 participants, MD: –3.03 [–3.48, –2.57], $I^2 = 0\%$).

Recurrence

Sixteen studies (H3, H6, H7, H9–H12, H17, H19, H25, H28, H29, H38, H42–H44) reported the rate of recurrence. Studies were grouped according to the time when follow-up assessment was conducted

(< 6 months or ≥ 6 months), and participants selected for assessment (all participants or those with an improvement). Meta-analysis was possible when oral CHM was compared with pharmacotherapy, and when oral CHM was used as an IM.

Oral Chinese herbal medicine alone

Six studies that evaluated oral CHM reported recurrence of signs and symptoms. Measurement of recurrence varied across studies based on which participants were assessed (all participants, or only those who received an improvement at the end of treatment) and when they were assessed (less than six months from end of treatment, or six months or greater) (Table 5.6). Oral CHM produced a greater reduction in the rate of recurrence within six months of the end of treatment when all participants were assessed (two studies; 91 participants, RR: 0.30 [0.13, 0.68], I^2 = 23%) and when only those who achieved improvement at the end of treatment were assessed (one study; 53 participants, RR: 0.70 [0.50, 0.97]). When the longer-term benefits of oral CHM were assessed, recurrence was lower in one study that

Table 5.6. Oral Chinese Herbal Medicine vs. Pharmacotherapy: Recurrence Rate

Assessment Criteria	No. of Studies (Participants)	Effect Size (RR [95% CI], I^2)	Included Studies
All participants, < 6 months from EoT	2 (91)	0.30 [0.13, 0.68]*, 23%	H9, H17
All participants, ≥ 6 months from EoT	1 (192)	0.62 [0.40, 0.95]*	H19
Cure/marked improvement/ improvement, < 6 months from EoT	1 (53)	0.70 [0.50, 0.97]*	H10
Cure/marked improvement/ improvement, ≥ 6 months from EoT	2 (73)	0.14 [0.01, 3.75], 81%	H3, H38

*Statistically significant.
Abbreviations: CI, confidence interval; EoT, end of treatment; RR, risk ratio.

assessed all participants, as opposed to only those who achieved an improvement.

Oral Chinese herbal medicine as an integrative medicine

Recurrence of atopic dermatitis was reported in ten studies (H6, H7, H11, H12, H25, H28, H29, H42–H44). One study (H28) presented data as a percentage, and another (H44) did not report the total number of people who were assessed for recurrence. Both studies were excluded from further analysis. The approach described earlier for oral CHM alone was used to categorise studies for analysis after considering the treatment in the comparator arm. Two meta-analyses were able to be conducted.

Oral CHM as an IM was more effective than pharmacotherapy alone at reducing the recurrence rate when all participants were assessed six months or more after the end of treatment (two studies; 165 participants, RR: 0.39 [0.23, 0.67], I^2 = 0%) (Table 5.7). Similar benefits were seen when those who achieved an improvement at the end of treatment were assessed within six months of the end of this

Table 5.7. Oral Chinese Herbal Medicine as an Integrative Medicine vs. Pharmacotherapy: Recurrence Rate

Assessment Criteria	No. of Studies (Participants)	Effect Size (RR [95% CI], I^2)	Included Studies
All participants, ≥ 6 months from EoT	2 (165)	0.39 [0.23, 0.67]*, 0%	H29, H42
Cure/marked improvement/ improvement, < 6 months from EoT	4 (297)	0.55 [0.41, 0.73]*, 0%	H7, H11, H12, H43
Cure/marked improvement/ improvement, ≥ 6 months from EoT	1 (34)	0.48 [0.27, 0.85]*, NA	H6

*Statistically significant.

Abbreviations: CI, confidence interval; EoT, end of treatment; NA, not applicable; RR, risk ratio.

treatment, and in a single study which assessed recurrence after 12 months.

Health-related Quality of Life

Health-related quality of life was less frequently measured than signs and symptoms of atopic dermatitis. Six studies (H20, H31, H35, H41, H49, H51) evaluated HRQoL using the Dermatology Life Quality Index (DLQI),[14] CDLQI[15] or a combination of both.

Oral Chinese herbal medicine alone

Four studies (H20, H41, H49, H51) reported HRQoL. One study that included children used the CDLQI (H49), and others used the DLQI (H41) or both CDLQI and DLQI (H20, H51). When an investigator-developed oral CHM formula was compared with epinastine, the DLQI score was higher at the end of treatment (indicating poorer HRQoL) in people who received oral CHM (60 participants, MD: 1.10 points [0.15, 2.05], H41). In children with atopic dermatitis, Hon *et al.* (2007) (H49) found that oral CHM improved HRQoL more than placebo on the CDLQI at 12 and 16 weeks. Data were presented graphically and were not able to be re-analysed.

Of the two studies that compared oral CHM with placebo plus pharmacotherapy, one study (H20) presented data that could be analysed. Both the CDLQI and DLQI were used to evaluate HRQoL, and the results were presented in aggregate. The investigator-developed formula was not statistically different to cetirizine, mometasone, plus placebo in improving HRQoL (20 participants, MD: −2.60 points [−7.36, 2.16]). One further study (H51) concluded that the change in HRQoL was greater with *Pei tu qing xin tang* 培土清心汤 at week 12 and week 36. Data for this study were not able to be analysed.

Oral Chinese herbal medicine as an integrative medicine

Of the two studies that evaluated the effect of oral CHM as an IM on HRQoL, one study (H31) did not report any results. Data were analysed for the second study (H35) that combined an investigator-developed oral CHM formula with mometasone furoate and levocetirizine. At the end of treatment, scores on the DLQI were 5.60 points lower in the treatment group, compared to the comparator group (90 participants, [–6.91, –4.29]).

Effective Rate

Effective rate was commonly reported, particularly in studies originating from China. Sixteen studies (H1, H9, H11, H15, H16, H22–H24, H27, H32, H36, H37, H39, H40, H43, H45) measured effective rate using the criteria set out in the 1994 guideline,[10] and four studies (H2, H7, H42, H46) used the 2002 guidleline[11] to assess effective rate. Results for these two guidelines were kept separate for analysis.

Oral Chinese herbal medicine alone

Effective rate was reported in seven studies (H9, H15, H22, H24, H27, H36, H37), all of which referred to the 1994 guideline.[10] The chance of achieving a 30%, or greater, improvement in atopic dermatitis signs and symptoms with oral CHM was 1.26 that of pharmacotherapy (seven studies; 503 participants, RR: 1.26 [1.09, 1.45]), $I^2 = 67\%$). Statistical heterogeneity was detected, and included studies were reviewed to conduct planned subgroup analyses. One of the seven studies was assessed as low risk of bias for sequence generation, and all studies provided treatment for one month or less. Subgroups for these factors were not able to be conducted. Similarly, there was no overlap in formulas across the studies. Subgroup analysis to explore potential sources of heterogeneity was not able to be conducted, and this result should be interpreted in light of the substantial statistical heterogeneity.

Oral Chinese herbal medicine as an integrative medicine

Thirteen studies evaluated the effect of oral CHM as an IM on effective rate according to the 1994 and 2002 guidelines.[10,11] In one study the results reported were incomplete, and data were not able to be re-analysed. When the 1994 guideline was followed, the chance of achieving a 30% or greater improvement in signs and symptoms was not different to pharmacotherapy (eight studies; 729 participants, RR: 1.23 [0.96, 1.58], I^2 = 96%) (Table 5.8). Statistical heterogeneity was considerable. Planned sensitivity and subgroup analyses were not able to be conducted, as treatment duration was similar across studies and only one study was assessed as low risk of bias for sequence generation. Furthermore, there was no overlap in formulas across the eight studies. The reliability of this finding remains uncertain. When the 2002 guideline was followed, the chance of achieving a 50%, or greater, improvement in signs and symptoms with oral CHM as an IM was 1.15 that of pharmacotherapy (four studies; 176 participants, RR: 1.15 [1.03, 1.30], I^2 = 50%) (Table 5.8).

Assessment Using Grading of Recommendations, Assessment, Development and Evaluation

Findings for important clinical questions were summarised using the Grading of Recommendations Assessment, Development and Evaluation (GRADE) approach. Consensus on items for inclusion was

Table 5.8. Oral Chinese Herbal Medicine as an Integrative Medicine vs. Pharmacotherapy: Effective Rate

Assessment Criteria	No. of Studies (Participants)	Effect Size (RR [95% CI], I^2)	Included Studies
1994 Guideline[10]	8 (729)	1.23 [0.96, 1.58], 96%	H1, H11, H16, H23, H32, H39, H43, H45
2002 Guideline[11]	4 (176)	1.15 [1.03, 1.30]*, 50%	H2, H7, H42, H46

*Statistically significant.
Abbreviations: CI, confidence interval; RR, risk ratio.

reached following the process described in Chapter 4. Outcomes selected were SCORAD,[9] itch severity, recurrence rate, DLQI or CDLQI as measures of HRQoL, and effective rate based on the criteria described in the 1994 guideline[10] (see Chapter 4 for details).

Oral CHM alone and oral CHM as an IM were selected for inclusion in summary-of-findings tables. Three comparators were selected: TCS, topical calcineurin inhibitors (TCI) and emollients. This translated to six possible summary-of-findings tables. However, for five of the six, there were no studies that evaluated these comparisons. Summary-of-findings tables were not able to be prepared for the following comparisons:

- Oral CHM alone vs. TCS.
- Oral CHM alone vs. TCI.
- Oral CHM alone vs. emollients.
- Oral CHM as an IM vs. TCI.
- Oral CHM as an IM vs. emollients.

In addition to the broad categories outlined above, several formulas included in Chapter 2 were rated as important for summary-of-findings tables. For the formulas *San xin dao chi yin* 三心导赤饮, *Xiao er hua shi tang* 小儿化湿汤, *Xiao er qi xing cha ke li* 小儿七星茶颗粒, *Shen ling bai zhu san (wan)* 参苓白术散 (丸), *Fang feng tong sheng wan* 防风通圣丸, *Run zao zhi yang jiao nang* 润燥止痒胶囊 and *Shi du qing jiao nang* 湿毒清胶囊, none of the included studies evaluated these treatments alone. Three formulas described in clinical textbooks and guidelines in Chapter 2 were evaluated in clinical studies. One study (H51) compared *Pei tu qing xin fang* 培土清心方 with mometasone (TCS) plus antihistamines; one study of modified *Dang gui yin* 加味当归饮 (H23) used an antihistamine as the comparator; three studies of *Xiao feng san* 消风散 (H5, H14, H21) used antihistamines as the comparator; and one compared *Xiao feng san* 消风散 with placebo (H47). All six studies were considered not eligible for GRADE assessment as they used comparators other than those selected through group consensus.

Table 5.9. GRADE: Oral Chinese Herbal Medicine as an Integrative Medicine vs. Topical Corticosteroids

Outcome (Treatment Duration)	Absolute Effect		Relative Effect (95% CI) No. of Participants (Studies)	Certainty of the Evidence GRADE
	With CHM	Without CHM		
Effective rate (4 wks)	**88** per 100 Difference: 12 more per 100 patients (95% CI: 3 fewer to 30 more per 100 patients)	**76** per 100	**RR 1.16** (0.96 to 1.40) 100 (1 RCT)	⊕⊕◯◯ LOW[a,b]

Note: (a) High risk of bias from blinding may influence results, and (b) Uncertainty in results is due to small sample size.

Abbreviations: CHM, Chinese herbal medicine; CI, confidence interval; GRADE, Grading of Recommendations Assessment, Development and Evaluation; RCT, randomised controlled trial; RR, risk ratio; wks, weeks.

Study reference: H16.

Oral Chinese herbal medicine as an integrative medicine vs. topical corticosteroids

One study (H16) compared oral CHM as an IM to TCS, with TCS alone. In this study, treatment was provided for four weeks. Based on low-certainty evidence, oral CHM as an IM was as effective as TCS alone, achieving 30%, or greater, improvement in atopic dermatitis signs and symptoms (Table 5.9). The study did not report adverse events.

Randomised Controlled Trial Evidence for Individual Oral Formulas

Several formulas or commercially available products were evaluated in two or more RCTs (see Table 5.1). Studies were reviewed to identify those that evaluated the same interventions and comparator types, and that reported on the same outcome measures. These studies were considered suitable for pooling, and meta-analyses conducted to determine the clinical evidence for formulas. Meta-analysis was possible for one commercial product: compound glycyrrhizin 复方甘草酸苷片.

Two studies (H29, H42) that evaluated compound glycyrrhizin 复方甘草酸苷片 as an IM to pharmacotherapy measured recurrence in all participants at six months. The risk of recurrence with compound glycyrrhizin 复方甘草酸苷片 as an IM was 0.39 that of pharmacotherapy alone (two studies; 165 participants, [0.23, 0.67], I^2 = 0%). Meta-analysis of the effective rate, according to the 2002 guideline,[11] showed that compound glycyrrhizin 复方甘草酸苷片 as an IM increased the chances of achieving a 50%, or greater, improvement in signs and symptoms (two studies; 139 participants, RR: 1.21 [1.03, 1.42], I^2 = 83%). Substantial statistical heterogeneity was detected but was not able to be explored due to the small number of studies. As both studies provided treatment for one month, and used antihistamines as co-interventions and comparators, these factors are unlikely to be the reason for heterogeneity.

Frequently Reported Orally Used Herbs in Meta-analyses Showing Favourable Effect

Oral Chinese herbal formulas have shown benefits for several outcomes, including SCORAD,[9] purititus severity, recurrence and effective rate. In order to understand which herbs may be contributing to the positive effects seen, further analysis of herb ingredients was undertaken. A selection of the most frequently used herbs is described in Table 5.10. All three meta-analyses of oral CHM for clinical signs indicated that oral CHM (alone or as an IM) could improve clinician-assessed signs. Sixteen studies were included in these analyses, and the most frequently used herb was *gan cao* 甘草. Results of patient-reported symptoms (pruritus) in three studies showed that four herbs were common to all studies: *yi yi ren* 薏苡仁, *bai zhu* 白术, *fu ling* 茯苓 and *tai zi shen* 太子参.

Eight studies were included in meta-analyses showing benefit of oral CHM for recurrence rate (Table 5.10). *Gan cao* 甘草 was

Table 5.10. Frequently Reported Orally Used Herbs in Meta-analyses Showing Favourable Effect

Herbs	Scientific Name	Frequency of Use
Clinical signs: 3 meta-analyses, 12 RCTs.		
Bai zhu 白术	*Atractylodes macrocephala* Koidz.	7
Bai xian pi 白鲜皮	*Dictamnus dasycarpus* Turcz	6
Dang gui 当归	*Angelica sinensis* (Oliv.) Diels	6
Fu ling 茯苓	*Poria cocos* (Schw.) Wolf	6
Gan cao 甘草	*Glycyrrhiza* spp.	6
Cang zhu 苍术	*Atractylodes* spp	5
Yi yi ren 薏苡仁	*Coix lacryma-jobi* L. var. mayuen (Roman.) Stapf	5
Patient-reported symptoms: 1 meta-analysis, 3 RCTs.		
Yi yi ren 薏苡仁	*Coix lacryma-jobi* L. var. mayuen (Roman.) Stapf	4
Bai zhu 白术	*Atractylodes macrocephala* Koidz.	3
Fu ling 茯苓	*Poria cocos* (Schw.) Wolf	3
Tai zi shen 太子参	*Pseudostellaria heterophylla* (Miq.) Pax ex Pax et Hoffm.	3
Recurrence: 2 meta-analyses, 8 RCTs.		
Gan cao 甘草	*Glycyrrhiza* spp.	8
Fu ling 茯苓	*Poria cocos* (Schw.) Wolf	6
Bai xian pi 白鲜皮	*Dictamnus dasycarpus* Turcz	4
Bai zhu 白术	*Atractylodes macrocephala* Koidz.	4
Chen pi 陈皮	*Citrus reticulata* Blanco	4
Huang qin 黄芩	*Scutellaria baicalensis* Georgi	4
Yi yi ren 薏苡仁	*Coix lacryma-jobi* L. var. mayuen (Roman.) Stapf	4
Effective rate: 2 meta-analyses, 11 RCTs.		
Gan cao 甘草	*Glycyrrhiza* spp.	6
Bai xian pi 白鲜皮	*Dictamnus dasycarpus* Turcz	5
Bai zhu 白术	*Atractylodes macrocephala* Koidz.	5
Fang feng 防风	*Saposhnikovia divaricata* (Turcz.) Schischk.	5
Dang gui 当归	*Angelica sinensis* (Oliv.) Diels	4
Fu ling 茯苓	*Poria cocos* (Schw.) Wolf	4

(Continued)

Table 5.10. (*Continued*)

Herbs	Scientific Name	Frequency of Use
Huang qin 黄芩	*Scutellaria baicalensis* Georgi	4
Ze xie 泽泻	*Alisma orientalis* (Sam.) Juzep.	4

Abbreviations: RCTs, randomised controlled trials.
Clinical signs: Refer to Tables 5.4, 5.5, and section 'SCOring of Atopic Dermatitis Index; Oral Chinese herbal medicine as an integrative medicine'. Patient-reported symptoms: See section 'Pruritus; Oral CHM alone'. Recurrence: Refer to Tables 5.6, 5.7. Effective rate: Section 'Effective rate; Oral CHM alone', Table 5.8.
Note: The use of some herbs may be restricted in some countries. Readers are advised to comply with relevant regulations.

used in all eight studies and *fu ling* 茯苓 was used in six studies. *Gan cao* 甘草 was also the most frequently used herb in studies which contributed to the positive effect seen on improving the effective rate.

There are many similarities in the most frequently used herbs in terms of clinical signs, patient-reported symptoms, recurrence and effective rate. The herbs described in Table 5.10 are also herbs that were used in oral CHM RCTs in general (see Table 5.2). This suggests that the formulas and herbs which may contribute to the positive effects seen are likely to be reflective of the formulas and herbs used more broadly for atopic dermatitis.

Safety of Oral Chinese Herbal Medicine in Randomised Controlled Trials

The safety of oral CM is an important factor that may influence treatment decisions. Adverse events were reported in 28 studies (1,042 participants in the intervention groups, 983 participants in comparator groups) (H3, H4, H9, H10, H14, H15, H17, H18, H20, H21, H23, H25–H27, H29–H31, H36, H39, H40, H41, H43, H45, H47–H51), with nine reporting that no adverse events occurred (H4, H14, H17, H18, H21, H23, H25, H39, H45). One study (H48) reported four cases of gastrointestinal upsets, two cases of transient dizziness, and one case each of increased hair loss and lichenoid eruption on the trunk. This study did not specify the group in which the adverse events occurred. A second study (H47) also did not report the group allocation of a case of transient increase in aspartate aminotransferase.

In studies that evaluated oral CHM alone, 111 adverse events were reported. Many were gastrointestinal in nature. Adverse events included 25 cases of abdominal discomfort or pain (with or without diarrhoea), 17 cases of upper respiratory tract infection, 11 cases of diarrhoea/loose stools, 12 cases of antibiotic use longer than three days, eight cases of a new rash, six episodes of asthma, five cases of topical or oral corticosteroid use, two hospitalisations (reasons not stated) and two cases of nausea. Six miscellaneous cases were reported in one study, including pustules, dizziness, bronchitis, ringworm, pompholyx and pneumonia; the study did not specify how many cases of each event. One case was reported of a diverse range of events, including anorexia, malaise, dizziness, headache, light-headedness, rhinitis, acne pustulosa, feverish thirst and dental caries. Laboratory adverse events included three cases of eosinophilia, and one case each of elevated glutamate pyruvate transaminase, immunoglobulin E, serum K and alanine aminotransferase, which returned to normal after ceasing treatment, and a decline in blood urea nitrogen. Fewer adverse events were reported when oral CHM was used as an IM. Adverse events included four cases of gastrointestinal discomfort and drowsiness, two cases of increased bowel movements, two cases of mild erythema with burning pain, and two cases of telangiectasia and hypopigmentation.

Ninety-two adverse events were reported with guideline-recommended treatments/placebo. Fewer adverse events in the comparator groups were gastrointestinal in nature. Twenty-two cases of dizziness and drowsiness were reported, as were seven cases of lethargy, four cases of drowsiness, and three cases of dizziness and fatigue. Dermatological events included six cases of mild erythema with burning or itching, three cases of mild oedema and erythema at the site of NB-UVB irradiation, five cases of new rash, three cases of telangiectasia and hypopigmentation, and one case each of pigmentation, itchy and burning sensation, and deepening of skin colour. Other adverse events included 15 upper respiratory tract infections, six cases of antibiotic use for more than three days, three episodes of asthma, two cases of diarrhoea/loose stools, two cases of abdominal pain and two hospitalisations for unspecified reasons. One case of topical or oral corticosteroid use was reported, and miscellaneous events in one study included pustules, appendectomy, menstrual disturbance and haematuria. Finally, there were an unspecified number of cases of drowsiness, dry mouth and indigestion.

Controlled Clinical Trials of Oral Chinese Herbal Medicine

Six controlled clinical trials (H52–H57) evaluated oral CHM. All six studies used a two-group parallel-arm design and were conducted in outpatient departments in China. The duration of atopic dermatitis in studies which reported this information ranged from two-and-a-half months to 19 years (H53). One study included only children (H56) and others included both adults and children (H52, H57). Two studies reported participant gender (H52, H57), and in both studies there were more males than females. In total, 402 people participated in the six studies. Treatment duration ranged from 14 days (H57) to two years (H55), and three studies (H52, H54, H56) provided treatment for four weeks. Four studies (H53–H56) reported conducting follow-up assessments after treatment had finished, which ranged from two months (H53, H54) to one year (H55).

One study (H52) reported using the CM syndrome of Blood deficiency and Wind-dry as an inclusion criterion. No other syndromes were reported. Two studies (H54, H57) compared investigator-developed oral CHM formulas with guideline-recommended treatments, and the remaining studies evaluated the combination of oral CHM with guideline-recommended treatments. Chinese herbal medicines were administered once (H52), twice (H54, H57) or three times per day (H53, H55, H56). Two studies used herb compounds/products including tanshinone from *dan shen* 丹参 and compound glycyrrhizin from *gan cao* 甘草. There was no overlap in formulas

Table 5.11. Frequently Reported Orally Used Herbs in Controlled Clinical Trials

Most Common Herbs	Scientific Name	Frequency of Use
Fang feng 防风	*Saposhnikovia divaricata* (Turcz.) Schischk.	4
Bai ji li 白蒺藜	*Tribulus terrestris* L.	2
Bai shao 白芍	*Paeonia lactiflora* Pall.	2
Bai zhu 白朮	*Atractylodes macrocephala* Koidz.	2
Dang gui 当归	*Angelica sinensis* (Oliv.) Diels	2
Fu ling 茯苓	*Poria cocos* (Schw.) Wolf	2
Sheng di huang 生地黄	*Rehmannia glutinosa* Libosch.	2

Note: The use of some herbs may be restricted in some countries. Readers are advised to comply with relevant regulations.

used across studies. The most frequently reported herb in the studies was *fang feng* 防风, used in four studies (Table 5.11). Treatments in comparator groups included antihistamines, topical and oral steroids, and topical non-steroidal anti-inflammatories.

Outcomes

Studies reported on a range of outcomes. Three studies (H53, H56, H57) reported on physician-assessed clinical signs, while none of the studies evaluated patient-reported symptoms. Three studies (H54–H56) reported on long-term control, one study (H57) reported on HRQoL using the DLQI[14] and one study (H52) reported on effective rate based on the 1994 guideline.[10] Four studies (H53–H56) reported on adverse events.

Clinical Signs

Three studies (H53, H56, H57) evaluated the effect of oral CHM on clinical signs. When clinical signs were evaluated using the SASSAD,[13] an investigator-developed oral CHM formula resulted in a lower score at the end of treatment compared with the antihistamine loratadine (56 participants, MD: –4.89 points [–7.54, –2.24], H57). Two studies that evaluated oral CHM as an IM found differing results. When compound glycyrrhizin tablets 复方甘草酸苷片 were combined with fexofenadine and butyl flufenamate ointment, no additional benefit was seen compared with fexofenadine and butyl flufenamate alone for the outcome SCORAD[9] (60 participants, MD: 1.82 points [–0.20, 3.84], H56). The combination of tanshinone tablets with cyproheptadine and TCS resulted in a lower score for symptoms and signs than cyproheptadine and TCS alone (64 participants, MD: –4.80 [–5.98, –3.62], H53). The details for assessing atopic dermatitis symptoms and signs were not reported, and the results of this study should be interpreted accordingly.

Recurrence

Three studies (H54–H56) evaluated recurrence, reporting the rate of recurrence at varying time points. Due to differences in the way in which recurrence was evaluated, the results were not able to be pooled for analysis. One study (H54) compared an investigator-developed oral CHM formula with prednisone. This study evaluated the rate of recurrence in people who achieved a 'cure' or 'most improved' at the end of treatment. The rate of recurrence between two and six months after the end of treatment with oral CHM alone was not statistically significant to prednisone (63 participants, RR: 0.55 [0.15, 2.00]).

Two studies evaluated oral CHM as an IM. One year after the end of treatment, the combination of *Yu ping fen* granules 玉屏风颗粒, loratadine and specific subcutaneous immunotherapy produced a statistically significant reduction in the recurrence rate in people who achieved a 'cure' (59 participants, RR: 0.16 [0.04, 0.66], H55). The recurrence was higher in people who received loratadine and specific subcutaneous immunotherapy alone. The second study found a reduction in the recurrence rate six months after the end of treatment in people who received compound glycyrrhizin tablets 复方甘草酸苷片 as an IM (48 participants, RR: 0.20 [0.05, 0.88], H56). No description was provided in relation to the participants who were assessed for follow-up.

Health-related Quality of Life

One study (H57) reported HRQoL using the DLQI.[14] An investigator-developed oral CHM formula produced a greater reduction, indicating better quality of life, at the end of treatment compared with loratadine alone (56 participants, MD: –4.94 points [–6.01, –3.87]).

Effective Rate

Effective rate was evaluated against the 1994 guideline[10] in one study (H52). The chance of achieving a 30%, or greater, improvement in symptoms was better with an investigator-developed oral CHM formula as an IM than with desloratadine plus desonide alone (72 participants, RR: 1.58 [1.19, 2.09]).

Safety of Oral Chinese Herbal Medicine in Controlled Clinical Trials

Four studies (H53–H56) reported on safety (140 participants in the intervention groups, 134 participants in the comparator groups), with no adverse events occurring in one study (H56). Adverse events with oral CHM alone included three cases of stomach discomfort and loss of appetite (H54). Two cases of mild rash with itch were reported when oral CHM was combined with cyproheptadine and TCS (H53). One study reported the total number of adverse events for both study groups (H55). Twelve cases of mild erythema and swelling at the immunotherapy injection site were reported, as were an unspecified number of cases of mild upper abdominal discomfort, nausea, loss of appetite and dizziness. Adverse events in the comparator groups included two cases of stomach discomfort, two cases of increased appetite, two cases of facial acne, and one case each of irregular menstruation and elevated blood pressure.

Non-controlled Studies of Oral Chinese Herbal Medicine

Thirty-six (H58–H93) non-controlled studies evaluated oral CHM. Twenty-seven studies (H58–H60, H62, H64–H66, H69–H74,

H76, H77, H79–H81, H83, H85, H87–H93) were case series, and nine studies (H61, H63, H67, H68, H75, H78, H82, H84, H86) were case reports. In total, 1,089 people were included in these studies.

Four studies (H58, H77, H80, H81) used CM syndromes as an inclusion criterion, including Blood deficiency and wind-dry syndrome, damp-heat syndrome, Spleen deficiency with dampness encumbrance, toxin invading the *ying* 营 level and stasis of Blood with *ying* 营 level heat. Fourteen studies (H59, H61–H63, H67, H68, H70, H75, H78, H82–H84, H86, H87) described CM syndromes that were used for treatment, with several studies reporting two or more syndromes, or two connected syndromes. The most frequently reported syndromes were Blood deficiency and wind-dry syndrome (H59, H75, H80), accumulation of damp-heat (H61, H62, H87), and damp-heat with wind/wind-heat with damp (H70, H75). Two syndromes were reported in two studies: Spleen deficiency and Blood dryness syndrome (H86, H87) and damp-heat toxin accumulation syndrome (H70, H82). Many syndromes were reported in only one study. These included accumulation of damp-heat with sluggish circulation of Blood (H61), *wei* 卫 level syndrome (H83), *qi* level syndrome (H83), *ying* 营 level syndrome (H83), Blood level syndrome (H83), damp-heat accumulation with Blood deficiency (H63), hyperactivity of Heart-fire and Liver-fire with damp-heat accumulating in the skin (H78), Spleen deficiency with wind excess syndrome (H86), Spleen *qi* impaired and prolonged disease involving the Kidney (H63), water-damp accumulation on the body surface with skin not being nourished (H84), weakness of the Spleen and Stomach leading to damp-heat accumulation (H68), damp-heat Blood dryness syndrome (H70), Spleen deficiency and Blood dryness syndrome (H86), syndrome of Lung Heat injuring *yin* (H67), syndrome of wind-dampness encumbering the skin (H82) and *yin* deficiency with Blood dryness (H62).

All 36 studies used at least one oral CHM product or formula, with several evaluating two or more formulas (H63, H66, H70, H75, H76, H82, H83, H87). As such, some studies may have used one herb twice, which increased its frequency in analyses. None of the included studies used CHM as an IM. Many of the studies used formulas which were developed by study investigators. *Xiao feng san* 消风散 was used in three studies (H75, H76, H83). The formula *Pei tu qing xin fang* 培土清心方 was named in four studies (H65, H69, H71, H72); however, only two studies (H65, H72) described the same herb ingredients. All other formulas were unique to individual studies. Among the 35 studies, *gan cao* 甘草 was the most frequently used herb (Table 5.12). *Glycyrrhiza* species were reported

Table 5.12.   Frequently Reported Orally Used Herbs in Non-controlled Studies

Most Common Herbs	Scientific Name	Frequency of Use
Gan cao 甘草	*Glycyrrhiza* spp	32
Sheng di huang 生地黄	*Rehmannia glutinosa* Libosch.	19
Dang gui 当归	*Angelica sinensis* (Oliv.) Diels	18
Chi shao 赤芍	*Paeonia* spp	16
Fang feng 防风	*Saposhnikovia divaricata* (Turcz.) Schischk.	15
Jing jie 荆芥	*Schizonepeta tenuifolia* Briq.	14
Huang qin 黄芩	*Scutellaria baicalensis* Georgi	13
Lian qiao 连翘	*Forsythia suspensa* (Thunb.) Vahl	13
Fu ling 茯苓	*Poria cocos* (Schw.) Wolf	12
Mu dan pi 牡丹皮	*Paeonia suffruticosa* Andr.	12
Yi yi ren 薏苡仁	*Coix lacryma-jobi* L. var. mayuen (Roman.) Stapf	12
Bai zhu 白术	*Atractylodes macrocephala* Koidz.	11
Cang zhu 苍术	*Atractylodes* spp	11
Huang bai 黄柏	*Phellodendron chinense* Schneid.	11
Di fu zi 地肤子	*Kochia scoparia* (L.) Schrad.	10
Jin yin hua 金银花	*Lonicera japonica* Thunb.	9
Bai xian pi 白鲜皮	*Dictamnus dasycarpus* Turcz.	9
Chan tui 蝉蜕	*Cryptotympana pustulata* Fabricius	9

Note: The use of some herbs may be restricted in some countries. Readers are advised to comply with relevant regulations.

32 times. Other frequently reported herbs included *sheng di huang* 生地黄 (19 uses), *dang gui* 当归 (18 uses), *chi shao* 赤芍 (16 uses) and *fang feng* 防风 (15 uses).

Safety of Oral Chinese Herbal Medicine in Non-controlled Studies

Eight non-controlled studies (H58, H66, H79, H80, H90–H93) involving 248 participants reported on adverse events, with three studies (H79, H90, H91) reporting no adverse events occurring during the study. Adverse events in the remaining studies included gastrointestinal complaints such as bloating, pain, stomach discomfort and diarrhoea (18 cases), three cases of rash, two cases of erythema and pain at the site of NB-UVB application, and one case each of suprapubic discomfort, skin pigmentation and increased bed-wetting in children.

Topical Chinese Herbal Medicine

Topical CHM was evaluated in 38 studies included in this review. These studies included 3,471 participants. Twenty-four studies were RCTs (H94–H117), four were CCTs (H118–H121) and 10 were non-controlled studies (H122–H131).

Randomised Controlled Trials of Topical Chinese Herbal Medicine

Topical CHM was evaluated in 24 RCTs involving 2,608 participants (H94–H117). One study was conducted in Taiwan (H116) and one in Iran (H117); all remaining studies were conducted in mainland China. All but two studies compared topical CHM with pharmacotherapy, placebo or a combination of the two. One three-arm study (H116) compared two different doses of CHM with placebo gel, and another three-arm study (H100) evaluated topical CHM alone and as an IM.

In studies that reported demographics of participants, there were more males than females (918 males compared to 746 females).

Some irregularities were noted in one study (H97), where the number of males and females in each group exceeded the number reported in each group. Participant age ranged from 10 months (H104) to 81 years (H115). Several studies (H94–H96, H111) focused on atopic dermatitis in children. There was a broad range in the duration of atopic dermatitis, from 4.3 days (H104) to 40 years (H115).

Treatment duration varied from seven days (H113) to eight weeks (H116). The majority of studies administered topical CHM for one month or less (21 studies; H94–H98, H100–H105, H107–H115, H117). Follow-up assessment was conducted in five studies (H100, H103–H105, H112). Assessments were made after four weeks (H105), two months (H100) or three months (H103, H104, H112). Loss to follow-up was reported in five studies (H96, H103, H109, H116, H117), with most studies reporting low rates of attrition (less than 10%). One study reported higher attrition, with 18 participants excluded from outcome analysis. Reasons for exclusion included necessity of systemic antibiotics, pregnancy/breastfeeding and unrelated skin disorders.

Six studies (H94–H98, H100) described using CM syndrome differentiation as an inclusion criterion for participating in the study. One study (H95) evaluated the same formula in three different syndromes: constitution of Spleen deficiency, constitution of dampness stagnation and constitution of Heart-fire hyperactivity. Damp-heat syndrome was described in four studies (H94, H96–H98), and Blood deficiency and wind-dryness in one study (H100).

Fourteen studies (H99–H102, H106, H108–H111, H113–H117) evaluated CHM alone, and 11 (H94–H98, H100, H103–H105, H107, H112) studies evaluated topical CHM as an IM. Many of the topical CHM formulas evaluated in these studies were investigator-developed. One formula, *Jin yu wai xi fang* 金鱼外洗方, was used in four studies by the same investigator (H94–H97), and a second formula, *Jin huang gao* 金黄膏, was used in two studies by the same investigator (H108, H109). One other formula was evaluated alone and as an IM in the same study (H100): *Fu fang liu lian pi ruan gao* 复方榴莲皮软膏, with the ingredients *liu lian pi* 榴莲皮, *ma chi xian* 马齿苋 and *bo he nao* 薄荷脑.

Table 5.13. Frequently Reported Topically Used Herbs in Randomised Controlled Trials

Most Common Herbs	Scientific Name	Frequency of Use
Huang bai 黄柏	*Phellodendron chinense* Schneid.	7
Ku shen 苦参	*Sophora flavescens* Ait.	6
Yu xing cao 鱼腥草	*Houttuynia cordata* Thunb.	5
Jin yin hua 金银花	*Lonicera japonica* Thunb.	4
Zi su ye 紫苏叶	*Perilla frutescens* (L.) Britt.	4
Wu wei zi 五味子	*Schisandra chinensis* (Turcz.) Baill.	4
Bo he 薄荷	*Mentha haplocalyx* Briq.	3
Da huang 大黄	*Rheum* spp	3
Di fu zi 地肤子	*Kochia scoparia* (L.) Schrad.	3
Gan cao 甘草	*Glycyrrhiza* spp	3
Huang qin 黄芩	*Scutellaria baicalensis* Georgi	3
Ma chi xian 马齿苋	*Portulaca oleracea* L.	3
Bai fan 白矾	Potassium aluminium sulfate	2
Bai xian pi 白鲜皮	*Dictamnus dasycarpus* Turcz.	2
Jiang huang 姜黄	*Curcuma longa* L.	2
Jing jie 荆芥	*Schizonepeta tenuifolia* Briq.	2
Liu lian pi 榴莲皮	*Durio* spp	2

Note: The use of some herbs may be restricted in some countries. Readers are advised to comply with relevant regulations.

Sixty-six different herbs were used in the 24 RCTs. The most frequently used herb in topical CHM studies was *huang bai* 黄柏, used in seven studies (Table 5.13). Other frequently used herbs included *ku shen* 苦参, *yu xing cao* 鱼腥草, *jin yin hua* 金银花 and *zi su ye* 紫苏叶.

All studies compared topical CHM with at least one guideline-recommended treatment or with placebo. Treatments included TCS, TCI, topical antibiotic/TCS combination treatments, antihistamines, antifungals and emollients. Two studies (H107, H117) compared topical CHM with placebo, one of which combined placebo with a topical antihistamine.

Risk of Bias

All studies were described using randomisation to allocate participants to groups; however, many lacked details on the method used (Table 5.14). Four studies used a random number table (H101, H103, H105, H112) and one used computer randomisation (H110). All five studies were judged as low risk for sequence generation. One study (H114) was judged to be at high risk of bias for sequence generation as the description appeared to suggest that sequential allocation was used. All studies were judged as unclear risk for allocation concealment as insufficient information was described.

One study (H114) blinded both participants and personnel to group allocation and was judged low risk for both domains. Three studies were judged as unclear risk for participant blinding as there was either insufficient information (H117) or no information about who was blinded to group allocation in the single blind design (H100, H102). Two studies (H116, H117) did not provide sufficient information to make a judgment for blinding of personnel. The majority of studies were judged as high risk for blinding of participants and personnel due to the nature of the interventions and comparators. Three studies (H110, H114, H116) blinded outcome assessors to group allocation and two studies (H102, H109) used objective outcome measures that were unlikely to be influenced by lack of blinding.

Table 5.14. Risk of Bias of Randomised Controlled Trials: Topical Chinese Herbal Medicine

Risk of Bias Domain	Low Risk *n* (%)	Unclear Risk *n* (%)	High Risk *n* (%)
Sequence generation	5 (20.8)	18 (75.0)	1 (4.2)
Allocation concealment	0 (0)	24 (100)	0 (0)
Blinding of participants	1 (4.2)	3 (12.5)	20 (83.3)
Blinding of personnel	1 (4.2)	2 (8.3)	21 (87.5)
Blinding of outcome assessors	5 (20.8)	19 (79.2)	0 (0)
Incomplete outcome data	22 (91.7)	1 (4.2)	1 (4.2)
Selective outcome reporting	0 (0)	24 (100)	0 (0)

One study (H117) did not describe reasons for loss to follow-up and no statistical method was used to account for missing data. This study was judged to be high risk of bias for incomplete outcome data. One study (H109) was judged as unclear risk as reasons for participant withdrawal were not provided. Other studies had no missing data, used methods to account for missing data or described reasons for withdrawal that were unlikely to relate to the treatment effect, and were judged low risk. None of the studies had published protocols, and all were judged as unclear risk for selective outcome reporting.

In addition to the potential sources of bias highlighted above, one study (H106) reported higher numbers of participants in the treatment group than in the control group (60 participants vs. 45 participants). The reason for the difference was not described. This may introduce some bias in the result and is worthy to note.

Outcomes

Not surprisingly, the most commonly reported outcomes were measures of clinical signs. The SCORAD[9] was reported in five studies and EASI[12] reported in four studies. Six studies reported on patient-reported symptoms and recurrence, two studies reported on HRQoL and eight studies reported on effective rate using the 1994[10] and 2002[11] guidelines. Whilst many studies reported these outcomes, not all studies presented data in a way that permitted re-analysis. Consequently, few meta-analyses were able to be conducted.

SCORing Atopic Dermatitis Index

Five studies (H95–H98, H100) evaluated the effect of topical CHM on SCORAD.[9] Meta-analysis was possible with studies that used topical CHM as an IM.

Topical Chinese herbal medicine alone

Results for people who received 28 days of treatment with the topical CHM formula *Fu fang liu lian pi ruan gao* 复方榴莲皮软膏 were not statistically different to mometasone furoate in terms of SCORAD (60 participants, MD: 1.47 points [–3.64, 6.58], H100).

Topical Chinese herbal medicine as an integrative medicine

Meta-analysis was possible for five studies that reported SCORAD (H95–H98, H100). Topical CHM as an IM resulted in a 3.06-point lower score at the end of treatment than pharmacotherapy alone (five studies; 664 participants, [–5.84, –0.29], $I^2 = 94\%$). Statistical heterogeneity was considerable. Subgroup analysis according to risk of bias assessment for the sequence generation domain was not possible as all studies were assessed as unclear risk. All five studies provided treatment for similar durations, and there was no overlap across studies in the topical CHM formulas. Planned subgroup analyses were not able to be conducted, and the result should be interpreted with caution.

One study (H95) included in the meta-analysis for SCORAD reported results according to syndrome differentiation that are worth highlighting. In this study, 30 patients with damp stagnation, Heart fire hyperactivity or Spleen deficiency were each allocated to the intervention and control group (180 participants in total). All participants received the same topical formula as an IM, an investigator-developed formula named *Jin yu wai xi fang* 金鱼外洗方 consisting of the herbs *yu xing cao* 鱼腥草, *jin yin hua* 金银花, *wu wei zi* 五味子, *huang bai* 黄柏 and *zi su ye* 紫苏叶. In this study, topical CHM as an IM was not superior to the antihistamine cyproheptadine hydrochloride in patients with damp stagnation (60 participants, MD: 0.00 [–1.86, 1.86]), Heart fire hyperactivity (60 participants, MD: –0.30 [–2.06, 1.46]) or Spleen deficiency (60 participants, MD: –0.40 [–2.36, 1.56]).

Eczema Area and Severity Index

Four studies (H103, H108, H111, H116) reported EASI,[12] with meta-analysis conducted for studies that compared topical CHM with pharmacotherapy.

Topical Chinese herbal medicine alone

Three studies of topical CHM alone (H108, H111, H116) measured clinical signs using EASI. Two of these compared topical CHM with pharmacotherapy and meta-analysis was conducted. Topical CHM was not significantly different to pharmacotherapy in reducing the EASI score (121 participants, MD: 0.21 points [–0.33, 0.74], I^2 = 0%, H111, H116). One study compared *Jin huang gao* 金黄膏 with the emollient Vaseline® (H108). No difference was seen between the two treatments in terms of EASI (90 participants, MD: –1.77 [–3.82, 0.28]).

Topical Chinese herbal medicine as an integrative medicine

One study (H103) reported an EASI score. After three weeks of treatment with an unnamed topical CHM formula as an IM, atopic dermatitis score was 6.30 points lower than with 0.03% tacrolimus ointment alone (63 participants, [–7.95, –4.45], H103).

Other Measures of Clinical Signs

Various other clinical signs were measured in included studies such as erythema, exudation and lichenification, TEWL, and Three-item Severity scale (TIS).[16] Eight studies (H94, H99, H102, H104, H110, H114, H116, H117) reported other measures of clinical signs.

Topical Chinese herbal medicine alone

Two studies described using the Rajka and Langeland scoring criteria[17] (H99) or overall assessment of clinical response (H117), but data were not able to be re-analysed. Results from single studies found benefits of topical CHM for some outcomes but not others. The formula *Fu yue kang xi ji* 肤悦康洗剂 produced a greater reduction in SASSAD score,[13] indicating clinical sign improvement, compared with loratadine plus 3% boric acid solution (115 participants, MD: –10.10 [–12.26, –7.94], H110). A reduction in papules was found with *Ding xiang luo le ru gao* 丁香罗勒乳膏, compared with halcinonide cream (80 participants,

MD: –0.27 [–0.47, –0.07], H114). The study also reported on lichenification; however, as no lichenification was noted in the halcinonide cream group, the effect of *Ding xiang luo le ru gao* 丁香罗勒乳膏 on this outcome was not able to be estimated.

One study (H102) reported on two measures of skin hydration. The water content of the stratum corneum was found to be improved with *Fu fang liu lian pi ruan gao* 复方榴莲皮软膏, compared with mometasone furoate cream (120 participants, MD: 9.29 [6.85, 11.73]). Transepidermal water loss was lower with topical CHM than mometasone furoate (120 participants, MD: –7.10 g/m²h [–8.82, –5.38]). Topical *Tzu-yun* ointment did not result in improvements in TIS.[16] The mean difference between groups at the end of treatment was –0.52 points (31 participants, [–1.64, 0.60], H116).

Topical Chinese herbal medicine as an integrative medicine

Two studies of topical CHM as an IM (H94, H104) reported on other measures of atopic dermatitis. Results from individual studies showed promising outcomes. Clinical signs and symptoms, including lesion severity and itch assessed using four-point scales, were reduced with topical CHM as an IM, compared to TCS alone (one study; 120 participants, MD: –1.00 [–1.12, –0.88], H104). One study of 120 participants (H94) evaluated three signs of atopic dermatitis: oedema, erythema and exudation. The investigator-developed formula as an IM reduced erythema (MD: –0.71 points [–0.86, –0.56]) and exudation (MD: –1.39 points [–1.48, –1.30]), but not oedema (MD: –0.16 [–0.34, 0.02]), compared with TCS alone.

Pruritus

Five studies (H94, H95, H97, H99, H114) measured itch severity. Meta-analysis was conducted with studies that used topical CHM as an IM.

Topical Chinese herbal medicine alone

Two studies (H99, H114) reported on itch severity, and data were able to be re-analysed for one study (H114). Itch severity on a four-point scale was 0.47 points lower with topical *Ding xiang luo le ru gao* 丁香罗勒乳膏 than with halcinonide cream (80 participants, [–0.74, –0.20]).

Topical Chinese herbal medicine as an integrative medicine

Three studies of topical CHM as an IM measured itch severity. Two studies (H95, H97) used a 10-cm VAS and the other (H94) did not specify how itch was measured. Data were pooled for meta-analysis using SMD. Topical CHM as an IM was not statistically different to pharmacotherapy in reducing itch severity (SMD: –0.63 [–1.47, 0.21], I^2 = 95%). Subgroup analysis was conducted according to the method used for measuring itch. When itch was evaluated using the 10-cm VAS, there was no difference between groups who received topical CHM as an IM and those who received pharmacotherapy, and statistical heterogeneity was eliminated (Table 5.15). In the study that did not specify the method of measurement, itch severity at the end of treatment with topical CHM as an IM was 4.00 points lower than pharmacotherapy.

One of the studies included in the meta-analysis in Table 5.15 (H95) reported itch scores according to CM syndrome differentiation. Itch severity was not statistically different between the treatment and comparator groups for syndromes: damp stagnation (60 participants,

Table 5.15. Topical Chinese Herbal Medicine as an Integrative Medicine vs. Pharmacotherapy: Itch Severity

Assessment Criteria	No. of Studies (Participants)	Effect Size (MD/ SMD [95% CI], I^2)	Included Studies
Itch severity (all)	3 (546)	SMD: –0.63 [–1.47, 0.21], 95%	H94, H95, H97
Itch severity (10-cm VAS)	2 (426)	MD: –0.29 [–0.62, 0.03], 0%	H95, H97
Itch severity (NS)	1 (120)	MD: –4.00 [–4.57, –3.43]* , NA	H94

*Statistically significant.
Abbreviations: CI, confidence interval; MD, mean difference; NS, not specified; SMD, standardised mean difference; VAS, visual analogue scale.

MD: –0.20 points [–1.08, 0.68]), Heart fire hyperactivity (60 participants, MD: –0.47 [–1.31, 0.37]), and Spleen deficiency (60 participants, MD: –0.20 [–1.10, 0.70]).

Other Patient-reported Symptoms

Sleep of patients with atopic dermatitis is often disturbed, and the extent of disturbance was measured in two studies (H95, H97). Sleep disturbance and itch severity were measured as a composite outcome in one study (H98). All three studies evaluated topical CHM as an IM. Two studies (H95, H97) reported on sleep disturbance using a 10-cm VAS. Sleep disturbance was reduced by 1.39 points when topical CHM was used as an IM (426 participants, [–1.85, –0.93], $I^2 = 57\%$). One of these studies (H95) reported results according to syndrome differentiation. Sleep disturbance was lower in participants with syndromes damp stagnation (60 participants, MD: –1.70 [–2.26, –1.14]) and Spleen deficiency (60 participants, MD: –1.87 [–2.72, –1.02]) who received treatment with topical CHM as an IM. In people with Heart fire hyperactivity, there was no statistical difference between the two groups (60 participants, MD: –0.56 [–1.32, 0.20]). One study (H98) reported on a composite measure of itch severity and sleep disturbance using a 10-cm VAS. This study found itch severity and sleep disturbance were rated 2.13 points lower with the formula *San wei qing re zhi yang xi ji* 三味清热止痒洗剂 as an IM than with TCS alone (64 participants, [–3.02, –1.24]).

Recurrence

The rate of recurrence was evaluated in six studies (H100, H103–H105, H112, H116). Differences were noted in the timing, participants were included in follow-up assessments and studies were kept separate for analysis. Meta-analysis was conducted where possible.

Topical Chinese herbal medicine alone

Two studies (H100, H116) reported on atopic dermatitis recurrence. Studies differed in the criteria used to assess recurrence and were not able to be pooled for analysis. In the thesis by Guo (2015) (H100), participants who achieved a clinical cure or met the criteria for 'most improved' were assessed for recurrence. The risk of recurrence two months after treatment was lower with *Fu fang liu lian pi ruan gao* 复方榴莲皮软膏 than with mometasone furoate (32 participants, RR: 0.32 [0.11, 0.92]). In the second study (H116), all participants were assessed four weeks after the end of treatment. The chance of recurrence within four weeks was not statistically different between those receiving *Tzu-yun* ointment and those receiving topical betamethasone valerate cream (31 participants, RR: 1.07 [0.17, 6.64]).

Topical Chinese herbal medicine as an integrative medicine

Recurrence of atopic dermatitis was reported in five studies (H100, H103–H105, H112) that used topical CHM as an IM. Topical CHM as an IM reduced the chance of recurrence within six months, compared with pharmacotherapy alone (Table 5.16). This effect was seen regardless of whether all participants were assessed (RR: 0.45 [0.25, 0.82], I^2 = 0%) or only those who achieved any improvement with treatment (RR: 0.27 [0.17, 0.44], I^2 = 0%).

Table 5.16. Topical Chinese Herbal Medicine as an Integrative Medicine vs. Pharmacotherapy: Recurrence Rate

Assessment Criteria	No. of Studies (Participants)	Effect Size (RR [95% CI], I^2)	Included Studies
All participants, < 6 months from EoT	2 (184)	0.45 [0.25, 0.82]*, 0	H103, H104
Cure/marked improvement/ improvement, <6 months from EoT	3 (149)	0.27 [0.17, 0.44]*, 0	H100, H105, H112

*Statistically significant.

Abbreviations: CI, confidence interval; EoT, end of treatment; RR, risk ratio.

Health-related Quality of Life

Health-related quality of life was not a commonly reported outcome. Two studies (one study with two treatment arms) measured the effect of topical CHM in participants with atopic dermatitis (H100, H103).

Topical Chinese herbal medicine alone

One study (H100) evaluated HRQoL using the DLQI[14] and CDLQI[15]. The results were presented in aggregate, as one mean and standard deviation for both questionnaires. *Fu fang liu lian pi ruan gao* 复方榴莲皮软膏 did not produce a statistically different result to mometasone furoate cream after 28 days of treatment (60 participants, MD: 1.24 [–0.38, 2.86]).

Topical Chinese herbal medicine as an integrative medicine

Two studies of topical CHM as an IM (H100, H103) reported on quality of life. One study (H103) used the DLQI, while the other used a combination of the DLQI and CDLQI. Studies were not pooled for analysis. When *Fu fang liu lian pi ruan gao* 复方榴莲皮软膏 was combined with mometasone furoate, there was no difference in scores on the CDLQI and DLQI at the end of treatment (60 participants, [–2.54, 0.48]; H100). An unnamed topical CHM formula as IM improved HRQoL on the DLQI by 1.77 points compared to tacrolimus (64 participants, [–2.20, –1.34]; H100).

Effective Rate

Eight studies (H99, H100, H103, H105, H106, H110, H111, H113) evaluated effective rate using either the 1994[10] or 2002[11] guidelines. Meta-analysis was conducted for studies that used topical CHM alone and those that combined topical CHM with guideline-recommended treatments.

Table 5.17. Topical Chinese Herbal Medicine vs. Pharmacotherapy: Effective Rate

Assessment criteria	No. of Studies (Participants)	Effect Size (RR [95% CI], I^2)	Included Studies
1994 Guideline[10]	4 (417)	1.02 [0.95, 1.10], 31%	H106, H110, H111, H113
2002 Guideline[11]	2 (210)	1.14 [0.67, 1.95], 91%	H99, H100

*Statistically significant.
Abbreviations: CI, confidence interval; RR, risk ratio.

Topical Chinese herbal medicine alone

Six studies reported the effective rate of topical CHM using either the 1994 guideline[10] (H106, H110, H111, H113) or the 2002 guideline[11] (H99, H100). Regardless of which guideline criteria were used to assess the clinical effect, topical CHM was not statistically different to guideline-recommended treatments (Table 5.17).

Topical Chinese herbal medicine as an integrative medicine

Two studies (H103, H105) reported effective rate using the 1994 guideline,[10] and one study (H100) referred to the 2002 guideline.[11] The chance of achieving a 30%, or greater, improvement in signs and symptoms with topical CHM as an IM was not statistically different to pharmacotherapy (two studies; 194 participants, RR: 1.05 [0.76, 1.45], $I^2 = 82\%$). Similarly, no difference was seen between the two groups in the chance of achieving a 50%, or greater, improvement (one study; 60 participants, RR: 0.89 [0.72, 1.10]).

Assessment Using Grading of Recommendations, Assessment, Development and Evaluation

The approach for selecting items for inclusion in summary-of-findings tables has been described under the section 'Oral Chinese Herbal Medicine.' Two comparisons that were considered important clinical questions were not evaluated in included studies: Topical

CHM alone vs. TCI and topical CHM as an IM vs. emollients. Furthermore, one study that evaluated a comparison of interest (topical vs. emollients) did not report on the outcomes selected. Finally, none of the three topical CHM formulas considered important by the expert group were evaluated in clinical studies (*Fu fang huang bai ye* 复方黄柏液, *Qing peng ru gao* 青鹏乳膏 and *Hei dou liu you ruan gao* 黑豆馏油软膏). Summary-of-findings tables were able to be prepared for three comparisons and are described below.

Topical Chinese Herbal Medicine vs. Topical Corticosteroids

The comparison of topical CHM with TCS was evaluated in six RCTs (H100, H102, H111, H113, H114, H116) that reported on selected outcomes. Topical CHM was not statistically different to TCS when atopic dermatitis signs were measured using SCORAD (moderate certainty evidence) (Table 5.18). Low-certainty evidence for topical CHM showed a greater reduction in itch severity measured on a four-point scale. Topical CHM was not different to TCS in terms of the effective rate based on low-certainty evidence. Recurrence rate was reported in two studies, but differences in criteria for measuring recurrence precluded pooling of results.

Adverse events were reported in all five studies. Adverse events in the intervention included burning/stinging sensation (four cases), stained clothes from ointment (three cases), red pimples and increased itching (one case). Adverse events in the comparator group included skin atrophy (seven cases), skin infections (five cases), telangiectasia (four cases), folliculitis-like rash (three cases), local mild discomfort (three cases), hormonal flushing (three cases), burning/stinging sensation and skin irritation (three cases), and pigmentation (two cases).

Topical Chinese Herbal Medicine as an Integrative Medicine vs. Topical Corticosteroids

Four studies (H98, H100, H104, H112) that reported on outcomes of interest compared topical CHM as an IM to topical corticosteroids.

Table 5.18. GRADE: Topical Chinese Herbal Medicine vs. Topical Corticosteroids

Outcome (Treatment Duration)	Absolute Effect		Relative Effect (95% CI) No. of Participants (Studies)	Certainty of the Evidence GRADE
	With CHM	**Without CHM**		
SCORAD (28 d)	**45.84** MD: 1.47 points higher (95% CI: 3.64 points lower to 6.58 points higher)	**44.37**	**MD: 1.47** (–3.64 to 6.58) 60 (1 RCT)	⊕⊕⊕◯ MODERATE[a]
Itch severity (4 wks)	**0.29** MD: 0.47 points lower (95% CI: 0.2 to 0.74 points lower)	**0.76**	**MD: –0.47**[*] (–0.74 to –0.20) 80 (1 RCT)	⊕⊕◯◯ LOW[a,b]
Effective rate: 1994 guideline (range 7 d to 4 wks)	**94** per 100 Difference: 1 fewer per 100 patients (95% CI: 7 fewer to 5 more per 100 patients)	**95** per 100	**RR: 0.99** (0.93 to 1.05) 265 (2 RCTs)	⊕⊕◯◯ LOW[a,c]

Note: (a) Uncertainty in results due to small sample siz; (b) Study at high risk of bias for sequence generation and allocation concealment; and (c) High risk of bias from blinding may influence results, downgrade one level.

*Statistically significant result.

Abbreviations: CHM, Chinese herbal medicine; CI, confidence intervals; d, days; GRADE, Grading of Recommendations Assessment, Development and Evaluation; MD, mean difference; RCT, randomised controlled trial; RR, risk ratio; SCORAD, SCORing Atopic Dermatitis Index; wks, weeks.

Study References: SCORAD: H100; Itch severity: H114; Effective rate: H111, H113.

Topical CHM as an IM reduced the SCORAD score and decreased the chance of recurrence, compared with TCS alone. The evidence for all outcomes was judged to be low, meaning we are less certain that the results reflect the true treatment effect (Table 5.19). Three studies (H98, H100, H112) reported adverse events. No adverse events were reported in the intervention group. An unspecified number of cases of mild drug dependence were reported in the comparator group.

Table 5.19. GRADE: Topical Chinese Herbal Medicine as an Integrative Medicine vs. Topical Corticosteroids

Outcome (Treatment Duration)	Absolute Effect		Relative Effect (95% CI) No. of Participants (Studies)	Certainty of the Evidence GRADE
	With CHM	Without CHM		
SCORAD (mean 4 wks)	25.83 MD: 3.92 points lower (95% CI: 2.02 to 5.82 points lower)	29.75	MD: −3.92* (−5.82 to −2.02) 124 (2 RCTs)	⊕⊕◯◯ LOW[a,b]
Recurrence[c] (mean 3 wks)	17 per 100 Difference: 60 fewer per 100 patients (95% CI: 34 to 70 fewer per 100 patients)	77 per 100	RR: 0.22* (0.09 to 0.56) 78 (2 RCTs)	⊕⊕◯◯ LOW[a,b]
Recurrence[d] (2 wks)	18 per 100 Difference: 22 fewer per 100 patients (95% CI: 6 to 30 fewer per 100 patients)	40 per 100	RR: 0.46* (0.25 to 0.85) 120 (1 RCT)	⊕⊕◯◯ LOW[a,b]

Note: (a) 'High' risk of bias from blinding may influence results; (b) Uncertainty in results due to small sample size; (c) Recurrence assessed for patients with cure/improvement, < 6 months from the end of treatment; and (d) Recurrence assessed for all patients, < 6 months from the end of treatment. *Statistically significant result.

Abbreviations: CHM, Chinese herbal medicine; CI, confidence intervals; GRADE, Grading of Recommendations Assessment, Development and Evaluation; MD, mean difference; RCT, randomised controlled trial; RR, risk ratio; SCORAD, SCORing Atopic Dermatitis Index; wks, weeks.

Study References: SCORAD: H98, H100; Recurrence[c]: H100, H112; Recurrence[d]: H104.

Topical Chinese Herbal Medicine as an Integrative Medicine vs. Topical Calcineurin Inhibitors

One study (H103) compared an unnamed topical CHM as an IM with TCI alone. The rate of recurrence within six months was low but was not statistically different to TCI alone (Table 5.20). Participants who received topical CHM as an IM fared better in terms of HRQoL

Table 5.20. GRADE: Topical Chinese Herbal Medicine as an Integrative Medicine vs. Topical Calcineurin Inhibitors

Outcome (Treatment Duration)	Absolute Effect		Relative Effect (95% CI) No. of Participants (Studies)	Certainty of the Evidence GRADE
	With CHM	**Without CHM**		
Recurrence[c] (3 wks)	**3** per 100 Difference: 6 fewer per 100 patients (95% CI: 9 fewer to 20 more patients per 100 patients)	**9** per 100	**RR: 0.35** (0.04 to 3.23) 64 (1 RCT)	⊕⊕○○ LOW[a,b]
DLQI (3 wks)	**4.76** MD: 1.77 points lower (95% CI: 1.34 to 2.2 points lower)	**6.53**	**MD: −1.77*** (−2.20 to −1.34) 64 (1 RCT)	⊕⊕○○ LOW[a,b]
Effective rate: 1994 guideline[10] (3 wks)	**77** per 100 Difference: 11 fewer per 100 patients (95% CI: 26 fewer to 10 more per 100 patients)	**88** per 100	**RR: 0.88** (0.7 to 1.11) 64 (1 RCT)	⊕⊕○○ LOW[a,b]

Note: (a) High risk of bias from blinding of participants and personnel, and unclear risk of blinding for outcome assessors may influence results; (b) Uncertainty in results due to small sample size; and (c) Recurrence assessed for all participants, < 6 months from the end of treatment. *Statistically significant result.

Abbreviations: CHM, Chinese herbal medicine; CI, confidence intervals; DLQI, Dermatology Life Quality Index; GRADE, Grading of Recommendations Assessment, Development and Evaluation; MD, mean difference; RCT, randomised controlled trial; RR, risk ratio; wks, weeks. Study References: Recurrence[c]: H103; DLQI: H103; Effective rate: H103.

on the DLQI than those who received TCI alone. The chance of achieving a 30%, or greater, improvement in symptoms (effective rate) was not statistically different between the two groups. The certainty of evidence for all three outcomes was low, meaning we are less certain that these results represent the true treatment effect.

The study reported more adverse events in the comparator group. Adverse events in the treatment group included burning sensation (two cases); dry skin (one case); and one other unspecified event. Adverse events in the topical calcineurin inhibitors group included burning sensation (three cases); pimples (two cases); one case each of itching and dry skin; and five other unspecified events.

Frequently Reported Topically Used Herbs in Meta-analyses Showing Favourable Effect

As described above, topical CHM was found to be effective in meta-analyses for the outcomes SCORAD and rate of recurrence. Additional evaluation of studies included in these meta-analyses was undertaken. Five studies were included in each meta-analysis for clinical signs and recurrence, and the most frequently used herbs are described in Table 5.21. Although the number of studies in each analysis was small, these herbs may provide promising leads for further studies or clinical practice. All of the herbs listed in Table 5.21 are found in the list of most frequently used herbs in all topical RCTs, albeit with lower frequency. These herbs are likely to be reflective of herbs generally used topically for atopic dermatitis.

Safety of Topical Chinese Herbal Medicine in Randomised Controlled Trials

Seventeen studies (H94–H96, H98, H100, H101, H103, H105–H107, H109, H111–H116) (878 participants in the treatment groups and 781 in the control groups) reported on adverse events, with six studies (H94–H96, H98, H106, H112) reporting no adverse events occurred. More adverse events were reported in the comparator group than in groups that received CHM (50 vs. 36, respectively). The 23 adverse events in people who received topical CHM alone were mostly dermatological. These included seven cases of increased burning and itching sensations, five cases of skin pigmentation and strong odour with topical CHM, four cases of burning or stinging

Table 5.21.   Frequently Reported Topically Used Herbs in Meta-analyses Showing Favourable Effect

Herbs	Scientific Name	Frequency of Use
Clinical signs: 1 meta-analysis, 5 RCTs.		
Wu wei zi 五味子	*Schisandra chinensis* (Turcz.) Baill.	3
Zi su ye 紫苏叶	*Perilla frutescens* (L.) Britt.	3
Jin yin hua 金银花	*Lonicera japonica* Thunb.	3
Yu xing cao 鱼腥草	*Houttuynia cordata* Thunb.	3
Huang bai 黄柏	*Phellodendron chinense* Schneid.	3
Recurrence: 1 meta-analysis, 5 RCTs.		
Ku shen 苦参	*Sophora flavescens* Ait.	3
Huang bai 黄柏	*Phellodendron chinense* Schneid.	2
Ma chi xian 马齿苋	*Portulaca oleracea* L.	2

Abbreviations: RCTs, randomised controlled trials.
Clinical signs: See 'SCOring of Atopic Dermatitis Index, Topical Chinese herbal medicine as Integrative Medicine'.
Recurrence: Refer to Table 5.16.
Note: The use of some herbs may be restricted in some countries. Readers are advised to comply with relevant regulations.

sensation, two cases of mild irritation, one case of skin flushing and one case of red pimples with increased itching. Five participants found the odour of the topical CHM intolerable and three participants reported that the ointment stained their clothes.

Among participants who received CHM as an IM, 13 adverse events were reported. These included four cases of local skin redness, four cases of mild gastrointestinal reactions, two cases of a burning sensation, and one case each of dry skin, itching, tingling and erythema. One adverse event of an unspecified nature was also reported. Fifty adverse events were reported with guideline-recommended treatments. These included 10 cases of a skin irritation/discomfort, burning or stinging, seven cases of skin atrophy, five gastrointestinal reactions, five cases of skin infections, four cases of telangiectasia, three cases of hormonal flushing, three cases of folliculitis-like rash, two cases of pigmentation, two cases of pimples, two cases of increased itching, and one case each of skin flushing and dry skin. An unspecified number of cases of mild drug dependence were reported, and five adverse events of an unspecified nature were also reported.

Controlled Clinical Trials of Topical Chinese Herbal Medicine

Four controlled clinical trials (H118–H121) evaluated topical CHM for atopic dermatitis. Three studies were conducted in China and were two-arm studies, and the fourth (H121) was conducted in Japan with three arms. Two hundred and thirty-seven people participated in these studies. There were more males than females included in the trials (130 males compared to 107 females). One study included both children and adults (H120), and the mean age reported in two studies suggested that participants were children (H118, H119). The mean age of participants in the fourth study was 15.6 years (H121). Treatment duration was short, ranging from three days (H118) to three weeks (H121). None of the studies reported follow-up assessment after treatment finished.

Chinese medicine syndromes were not described in the included studies. Topical CHM formulas were developed by study investigators. No single formula was evaluated in more than one study. Interestingly, the herbal ingredients were unique to each study, and no herbs were used in two or more studies. Topical CHMs were compared with topical pharmacotherapy, including TCS and moisturisers (H118, H119), petrolatum or saline (H121) or no treatment in a study that used a left-right control design (H120).

Outcomes

Two studies each reported on clinician assessed signs (H120, H121), effective rate (H118, H119) and adverse events (H120, H121). One study reported on patient-reported symptoms (H120). None of the studies that evaluated topical CHM reported on long-term control or HRQoL.

Clinical Signs

Of the two studies that reported clinical signs of atopic dermatitis, only one (H120) presented data in a way which permitted re-analysis. In this study, four items were scored on a four-point scale: erythema, papules, infiltration hypertrophy and dryness. The maximum score, indicating worse disease, was 12 points. Compared with no treatment, the topical CHM *Wei nuo na rou run bao shi shuang* 薇诺娜柔润保湿霜, containing extract of purslane and avocado, significantly reduced atopic dermatitis severity (80 participants, MD: –2.40 [–2.72, –2.08]).

Patient-reported Symptoms

The study that evaluated clinical signs also evaluated patient-reported symptoms (H120). The same four items assessed by clinicians were also assessed by patients. *Wei nuo na rou run bao shi shuang* 薇诺娜柔润保湿霜 significantly reduced the self-assessed severity of symptoms by 2.10 points, compared with no treatment (80 participants, [–2.46, –1.74]).

Effective Rate

Two studies (H118, H119) reported effective rate using the 1994 guidelines,[10] and meta-analysis was able to be conducted. The application of topical CHM did not significantly increase the chance of achieving a 30%, or greater, improvement in signs and symptoms, compared to the combination of TCS and moisturisers (190 participants, RR: 1.33 [0.3, 2.80], $I^2 = 94\%$).

Safety of Topical Chinese Herbal Medicine in Controlled Clinical Trials

Adverse events were reported in two studies (H120, H121) (96 participants in the treatment groups, 94 participants in the control groups), with one study (H121) reporting that no adverse events occurred. Findings from one study showed one case of local itching and one case of a burning sensation among people who received topical CHM.

Non-controlled Studies of Topical Chinese Herbal Medicine

Fewer non-controlled studies evaluated topical CHM than oral CHM, with ten studies (H122–H131) being included in this section. One study was a case report (H131) and the rest were case series. Six hundred and nineteen people participated in the ten studies. Two studies (H122, H125) reported the CM syndromes used to guide treatment. Each study described two syndromes: damp-heat syndrome and Blood deficiency with wind-dryness syndrome (H122), Spleen deficiency with Blood dryness syndrome and *yin* deficiency with Blood dryness (H125). There was no overlap between the two studies in CM syndromes.

Three studies combined topical CHM with conventional medicine treatments such as tacrolimus ointment (H125), desonide cream (H129) and other atopic dermatitis medication (H131). Many of the formulas and products evaluated were investigator-developed. Two studies used topical CHMs that were not developed by the study investigators. These studies evaluated *Dan pi fen ruan gao* 丹皮酚软膏 (H129) and topical application of bitter melon (*ku gua* 苦瓜) (H131). There was little overlap in herbs used across studies (Table 5.22).

Safety of Topical Chinese Herbal Medicine in Non-controlled Studies

Five studies (H125, H127–H130), including 386 participants, reported on adverse events. In one study (H130), no adverse events occurred. Adverse events were mostly dermatological in nature (26 cases), and included itching, tingling, erythema, dryness, desquamation and aggravation of rash. In addition, two cases of elevated red blood cells in urine occurred which resolved spontaneously.

Table 5.22. Frequently Reported Topically Used Herbs in Non-controlled Studies

Most Common Herbs	Scientific Name	Frequency of Use
Bai xian pi 白鲜皮	*Dictamnus dasycarpus* Turcz.	3
Cang zhu 苍术	*Atractylodes* spp	3
Da huang 大黄	*Rheum* spp	3
Ku shen 苦参	*Sophora flavescens* Ait.	3
Dang gui 当归	*Angelica sinensis* (Oliv.) Diels	2
Di fu zi 地肤子	*Kochia scoparia* (L.) Schrad.	2
Fang feng 防风	*Saposhnikovia divaricata* (Turcz.) Schischk.	2
Huang qin 黄芩	*Scutellaria baicalensis* Georgi	2
Jing jie 荆芥	*Schizonepeta tenuifolia* Briq.	2
Ma chi xian 马齿苋	*Portulaca oleracea* L.	2
She chuang zi 蛇床子	*Cnidium monnieri* (L.) Cuss.	2

Note: The use of some herbs may be restricted in some countries. Readers are advised to comply with relevant regulations.

Oral Plus Topical Chinese Herbal Medicine

Thirty-three studies, involving 2,607 participants, evaluated the combination of oral with topical CHM. Eighteen of these were RCTs (H20, H51, H132–H147), one was a non-randomised CCT (H148) and 14 were non-controlled studies (H149–H162).

Randomised Controlled Trials of Oral Plus Topical Chinese Herbal Medicine

More than 1,800 people (1,859) participated in the 18 included RCTs. Seventeen studies were conducted in mainland China and one study (H143) was conducted in Hong Kong. Most trials were conducted in hospital outpatient departments, with two (H145, H146) conducted in both inpatient and outpatient departments. All but two studies used a two-arm parallel group design; two studies included three arms (H20, H51). In studies that reported disease duration, participants had lived with atopic dermatitis for between five days (H136) and 40 years (H143). Several studies (H132, H133, H140, H141, H147) focused on children with atopic dermatitis, while others included both adults and children. Participant age ranged from less than 12 months (H140) to 80 years (H144). In studies that reported mean age of participants, the median was 14 years. There were more males than females in the studies (853 males compared to 787 females).

Treatment duration ranged from 15 days (H136) to three months (12 weeks) (H20, H51, H133), with the majority of studies providing treatment for four or eight weeks. Eight RCTs conducted follow-up assessments after treatment had finished, occurring at approximately three (H134, H146), six (H20, H51, H137, H138) and 12 months (H136, H144). Four studies (H51, H134, H138, H139) reported loss to follow-up, with a similar number of participants withdrawing across the groups.

Chinese medicine syndrome differentiation was used as an inclusion criterion and to guide treatment. In the seven studies that used syndrome differentiation as an inclusion criterion, the most frequently reported syndrome was Blood deficiency and wind-dryness, reported in three studies (H137–H139). There was no overlap across studies in other syndromes, which included damp-heat accumulation (H133), Spleen deficiency with dampness retention (H133), wind-dampness encumbering the skin (H134), Spleen deficiency and Blood dryness (H145) and damp-heat (H146). In six studies that used syndrome differentiation to guide treatment, three syndromes were reported in two studies: wind-dampness encumbering skin (H135, H144), Blood deficiency and wind-dryness (H135, H144) and damp-heat/damp-heat accumulation (H140, H141). Other syndromes included Spleen deficiency with dampness retention (H140), Spleen deficiency and Blood dryness (H141), foetal heat (H142), Spleen dampness (H142), *yin* deficiency and Blood dryness (H142), relative predominance of Heart-fire (H51) and relative predominance of Spleen deficiency (H51).

All but one of the RCTs evaluated the combination of oral and topical CHM alone. The RCT which used oral plus topical CHM as an IM combined CHM with loratadine and vitamin C (H142). Many of the formulas used orally or topically were either not named or were developed by study investigators. One formula was used in two studies: *Chu shi wei ling tang* 除湿胃苓汤 (H135, H142). There was no overlap across studies in other formulas.

Seventy-four different herbs were used in RCTs of oral plus topical CHM. Not surprisingly, the most frequently used herbs were a mix of those commonly reported in RCTs of oral and topical CHM (Tables 5.2 and 5.13). The most frequently reported herbs, used in 15 studies each, were *fu ling* 茯苓 and *gan cao* 甘草. Other frequently used herbs included *bai xian pi* 白鲜皮, *sheng di huang* 生地黄 and *yi yi ren* 薏苡仁 (Table 5.23).

Table 5.23. Frequently Reported Orally and Topically Used Herbs in Randomised Controlled Trials

Most Common Herbs	Scientific Name	Frequency of Use
Fu ling 茯苓	*Poria cocos* (Schw.) Wolf	15
Gan cao 甘草	*Glycyrrhiza* spp	15
Bai xian pi 白鲜皮	*Dictamnus dasycarpus* Turcz.	12
Sheng di huang 生地黄	*Rehmannia glutinosa* Libosch.	11
Yi yi ren 薏苡仁	*Coix lacryma-jobi* L. var. mayuen (Roman.) Stapf	11
Dang gui 当归	*Angelica sinensis* (Oliv.) Diels	9
Bai zhu 白术	*Atractylodes macrocephala* Koidz.	8
Long gu 龙骨	Fossilised bone	8
Jin yin hua 金银花	*Lonicera japonica* Thunb.	7
Mu li 牡蛎	*Ostrea* spp	7
Ci ji li 刺蒺藜 (*bai ji li* 白蒺藜)	*Tribulus terrestris* L.	6 (4)
Di fu zi 地肤子	*Kochia scoparia* (L.) Schrad.	6
Ze xie 泽泻	*Alisma orientalis* (Sam.) Juzep.	6
Bai shao 白芍	*Paeonia lactiflora* Pall.	5
Cang zhu 苍术	*Atractylodes* spp	5
Dan zhu ye 淡竹叶	*Lophatherum gracile* Brongn.	5
Gu sui bu 骨碎补	*Drynaria fortunei* (Kunze) J. Sm.	5
Huang bai 黄柏	*Phellodendron chinense* Schneid.	5
Ku shen 苦参	*Sophora flavescens* Ait.	5

Note: The use of some herbs may be restricted in some countries. Readers are advised to comply with relevant regulations.

Comparators included at least one guideline-recommended pharmacotherapy. These included TCS, oral antihistamines and boric acid solution. Some studies combined guideline-recommended treatments with various other treatments, including vitamin C (H135, H141, H142), oral transfer factor (H141) and topical creams comprising triamcinolone acetonide, neomycin sulfate and miconazole nitrate (H132). Vitamin C is not recommended in clinical guidelines but may be used as adjuvant therapy to reduce exudation in the acute stage. Two studies (H20, H51) combined placebo with pharmacotherapies.

Risk of Bias

Potential sources of bias were assessed (Table 5.24). All studies were described as being randomised. Five studies (H51, H134, H138, H139, H145) described using a random number table for group allocation and were judged as low risk of bias. One study (H51) used central randomisation controlled by an independent investigator and was judged low risk for group allocation. Due to the nature of the interventions and comparators, it was not possible to blind participants to group allocation. One study (H51) reported that their study code and the drugs used by patients were

Table 5.24. Risk of Bias of Randomised Controlled Trials: Oral plus Topical Chinese Herbal Medicine

Risk of Bias Domain	Low Risk *n* (%)	Unclear Risk *n* (%)	High Risk *n* (%)
Sequence generation	5 (27.8)	13 (72.2)	0 (0)
Allocation concealment	1 (5.6)	17 (94.4)	0 (0)
Blinding of participants	0 (0)	0 (0)	18 (100)
Blinding of personnel	1 (5.6)	0 (0)	17 (94.4)
Blinding of outcome assessors	1 (5.6)	17 (94.4)	0 (0)
Incomplete outcome data	17 (88.9)	1 (5.6)	0 (0)
Selective outcome reporting	1 (5.6)	16 (88.8)	1 (5.6)

concealed from study investigators, and participants were asked not to reveal the allocated treatment. Blinding was assessed in this study and was judged to be effective. This study posed low risk of bias. All remaining studies were at high risk of bias for blinding of personnel. In relation to outcome assessment, one study had an independent assessor evaluate outcomes and was judged as low risk (H51). One study reported that a third party assessed the outcomes. This study posed unclear risk of bias, as did the remaining studies for which there was insufficient information reported.

Twelve studies (H20, H132, H133, H135–H137, H140–H144, H146) reported no missing data, posing low risk. A further five studies reported participant withdrawal but were judged low risk as the numbers were balanced across groups (H51, H134, H139), and/or because appropriate statistical methods were used to analyse data (H51, H138, H147). One study (H145) was assessed as posing unclear risk for incomplete outcome data because the reasons for withdrawal were not reported. One study (H51) had published a trial protocol and reported on all pre-specified outcomes. This study was assessed as low risk of bias. One study (H146) was judged as high risk for selective outcome reporting as outcomes described in the methods were not reported.

While other potential sources of bias were not assessed for all studies, two RCTs had potential sources of bias that are worth describing. The study by Fu (2000) (H136) had a large difference in the number of participants in the two arms (160 people in the intervention arm, 100 people in the comparator group). There was no description of the randomisation ratio, nor was any reason for the difference described. This may contribute to overestimation of the treatment effect. The study by Li, Cheng and Bai (2013) (H140) included infants and children, many of whom were under one month of age. In this study, children in the comparator group received fluocinolone acetate cream, which may be considered a strong treatment for infants. Furthermore, the use of oral CHM in children under one month of age is unusual; however, the authors reported no adverse events.

Outcomes

All studies reported on at least one of the pre-specified outcomes. The most frequently reported outcomes were adverse events (14 studies), followed by clinical signs of atopic dermatitis (10 studies). Seven studies evaluated disease severity using SCORAD,[9] two used EASI[12] and one study used an investigator-developed assessment of severity. Seven studies evaluated patient-reported symptoms, including four that measured itch severity, two that evaluated the composite measure of itch severity plus sleep score and one study that evaluated patient self-assessment. Four studies reported recurrence rate, four studies reported on HRQoL with three using a combination of the DLQI[14] and CDLQI[15] and six studies evaluated effective rate.

SCORing Atopic Dermatitis Index

The SCORAD was reported in seven studies (H20, H51, H134, H137, H138, H146, H147). Five studies compared oral plus topical CHM with guideline-recommended treatments at the end of eight weeks, and meta-analysis was conducted (Table 5.25). The combination of oral plus topical CHM reduced clinical signs by 4.82 points (356 participants, [–8.90, –0.73], $I^2 = 69\%$). Statistical heterogeneity was detected and was unable to be reduced with sensitivity analyses of studies assessed as low risk of bias for sequence generation. As all studies provided treatment for eight weeks, it was not possible to conduct subgroup analysis for treatment duration.

Table 5.25. Oral Plus Topical Chinese Herbal Medicine vs. Pharmacotherapy: SCORing Atopic Dermatitis Index

Studies	No. of Studies (Participants)	Effect Size (MD [95% CI], I^2)	Included Studies
All studies	5 (356)	–4.82 [–8.90, –0.73]*, 69%	H134, H137, H138, H146, H147
Low risk of bias for sequence generation	2 (160)	–4.67 [–13.41, 4.07], 80%	H134, H138

*Statistically significant.

Abbreviations: CI, confidence interval; m, months.

Two studies (H20, H51) compared SCORAD results for oral plus topical CHM and pharmacotherapy plus placebo. Data were able to be re-analysed for the study by Rao (2010) (H20). Oral plus topical CHM reduced SCORAD score by 11.05 points ([−14.44, −7.66]) compared with pharmacotherapy and placebo. Results from Liu *et al.* (2015) (H51) indicated that oral plus topical CHM produced a greater reduction in SCORAD at 28 weeks and 36 weeks, compared with placebo plus pharmacotherapy.

Eczema Area and Severity Index

Two studies (H139, H145) used EASI to assess clinical signs. After four weeks of treatment, the EASI score was 1.30 points lower among those who received oral plus topical CHM than those who received pharma-cotherapy (146 participants, [−2.48, −0.11], $I^2 = 59\%$). Subgroup analysis to explore the substantial statistical heterogeneity was not able to be conducted due to the small number of included studies.

Other Measures of Clinical Signs

Investigators of one study (H141) developed their own method to assess the severity of skin lesions and itching. The details for scoring were not available. In this study an investigator-developed formula, used both orally and topically for one month, produced a greater improvement in skin lesions and pruritus compared with chlorpheniramine, vitamin C and oral transfer factor (MD: −1.10 points [−1.12, −1.08]).

Pruritus

Four studies (H137, H139, H141, H145) that evaluated oral plus topi-cal CHM alone measured itch severity using a 10-cm VAS or a four-point scale. Due to the different methods for measuring itch sever-ity, the overall meta-analysis was conducted using SMD (Table 5.26). Compared with pharmacotherapy, the combination of oral plus topical CHM produced a significant improvement in itch severity (SMD: −2.42 [−4.08, −0.76]). Statistical heterogeneity was considerable ($I^2 = 97\%$), and sensitivity analysis of two studies with low risk of bias for sequence

Table 5.26. Oral plus Topical Chinese Herbal Medicine vs. Pharmacotherapy: Itch Severity

Studies	No. of Studies (Participants)	Effect Size (MD/ SMD [95% CI], I²)	Included Studies
All studies	4 (287)	SMD: –2.42 [–4.08, –0.76]*, 97%	H137, H139, H141, H145
4-week treatment duration	3 (207)	SMD: –3.61 [–6.20, –1.02]*, 98%	H139, H141, H145
Low risk of bias for sequence generation	2 (147)	SMD: –0.57 [–0.90, –0.24]*, 0%	H139, H145
10-cm visual analogue scale	2 (162)	MD: –0.50 [–1.09, 0.09], 21%	H137, H145
4-point scale	2 (125)	MD: –0.56 [–0.70, –0.42]*, 32%	H139, H141

* Statistically significant. Abbreviations: CI, confidence interval; MD, mean difference; SMD, standardised mean difference.

generation was able to eliminate this whilst maintaining the treatment effect. Analysis of these two studies provides the best evidence for oral plus topical CHM in reducing itch. Interestingly, when study results were analysed according to the method used to score itch (10-cm VAS or four-point scale), statistical heterogeneity was also reduced. In studies where the 10-cm VAS was used, the effect of CHM was no longer statistically significant. This may relate to greater possibility for variation in results — possible result ranges from 0 to 10 as opposed to 0 to 4; however, variation would have been taken into account when using SMD for analysis. The reasons why one method produced a statistically significant result while the other did not are unclear.

Other Patient-reported Symptoms

Two studies (H134, H138) combined assessment of itch with assessment of sleep loss. Assessments for both items were made using a 10-cm VAS, with the possible score ranging from zero to 20. Meta-analysis showed no statistical difference in itch and sleep loss between people who received oral plus topical CHM alone, and those who received pharmacotherapy (160 participants, MD: –0.66 [–1.83, 0.50], I² = 0%).

One study (H51) used patient self-assessment on a VAS from 0 to 10, where a lower score indicated worse severity. Data were not presented in a way that permitted re-analysis. The authors reported that people who received oral plus topical CHM achieved a better self-assessment of their symptoms than people who received pharmacotherapy plus placebo at 20, 28 and 36 weeks after the start of treatment.

Recurrence

Recurrence of atopic dermatitis was evaluated in four studies (H134, H136–H138), all of which evaluated oral plus topical CHM alone. Studies were grouped according to the criteria for selecting participants to assess for recurrence (all participants, or those with an improvement at end of treatment) and the time at which recurrence was assessed (less than six months, or six months or greater). None of the four studies evaluated all participants who were randomised. Three studies (H136–H138) evaluated recurrence at six months or greater in participants with sign and symptom improvement at the end of treatment. In these studies, the risk of recurrence was lower in people who received oral plus topical CHM, compared with pharmacotherapy (281 participants, RR: 0.44 [0.35, 0.56], $I^2 = 0\%$). One study (H134) evaluated recurrence after three months in people who achieved an improvement in symptoms. An investigator-developed oral plus topical CHM reduced the risk of recurrence, compared to pharmacotherapy (47 participants, RR: 0.34 [0.14, 0.84]). The same study also reported time to recurrence, with people who received oral plus topical CHM having 24.63 more days before recurrence than people who received pharmacotherapy alone ([20.84, 28.42]).

Health-related Quality of Life

Four studies (H20, H51, H137, H138) reported HRQoL. All four studies used oral plus topical CHM alone as the intervention. Data were able to be analysed for three studies (H20, H137, H138). One study (H137) did not report the outcome tool used, one (H20) used both the DLQI[14] and CDLQI[15] and the third (H138) used DLQI, CDLQI and the Infant Dermatology Life Quality Index (IDLQI)[18] according to the age of individual participants. Meta-analysis was conducted using SMD for pooled data and MD for individual studies.

When oral plus topical CHM was compared with pharmaco-therapy, no statistically significant difference was detected (two studies; 142 participants, SMD: −0.13 [−0.46, 0.20], I² = 0%, H137, H138). Results from one study showed similar results on the DLQI and CDLQI when investigator-developed oral plus topical CHM was compared with placebo, cetirizine and mometasone furoate (20 participants, MD: −1.70 [−6.01, 2.61]). The final study (H51) evaluated quality of life using the DLQI and CDLQI. The authors concluded that quality of life was superior with oral plus topical CHM at 36 weeks compared with placebo plus mometasone furoate and loratadine.

Effective Rate

Effective rate was evaluated in seven studies (H132, H135, H141–H145). One study measured the effective rate using the criteria from the 2002 guideline,[11] and all other studies used the 1994 guideline criteria.[10]

Oral Chinese herbal medicine alone

Six studies (H132, H135, H141, H143–H145) that investigated oral plus topical CHM included effective rate using the 1994[10] and 2002[11] guidelines. Results were not reported in one study (H141). In the five studies that compared oral plus topical CHM with phar-macotherapy, the chance of achieving an improvement in signs and symptoms was not statistically different. This finding was seen with both the 1994 guideline criteria (four studies; 423 participants, RR: 1.25 [0.89, 1.76], I² = 94%, H132, H135, H143, H144) and the 2002 guideline criteria (one study; 82 participants, RR: 1.16 [0.90, 1.49], H145).

Oral Chinese herbal medicine as an integrative medicine

One study (H142) used oral plus topical CHM as an IM. In this study, the chance of achieving a 30%, or greater, improvement was higher with the combination of modified *Chu shi wei ling tang* 除湿胃苓汤加减 (oral), modified *Dang gui yin zi* 当归饮子加减 (oral) and *Shi zhen san* 湿疹散 (topical) than with loratadine and vitamin C (100 participants, RR: 1.21, [1.02, 1.44]).

Assessment Using Grading of Recommendations, Assessment, Development and Evaluation

The approach for selecting content for summary-of-findings tables has been described in the section 'Oral Chinese Herbal Medicine.' Few studies evaluated the comparisons selected with the outcomes agreed upon by group consensus. Summary-of-findings tables were not able to be prepared for oral plus topical CHM alone vs. TCI or emollients, and no summary-of-findings tables could be prepared for oral plus topical CHM as an IM.

Oral Plus Topical Chinese Herbal Medicine vs. Topical Corticosteroids

One study (H140) evaluated the comparison of oral plus topical CHM vs. TCS. The study reported on adverse events, with none occurring during the study.

Frequently Reported Orally and Topically Used Herbs in Meta-analyses Showing Favourable Effect

The combination of oral plus topical CHM was found to reduce atopic dermatitis signs and itch severity, and to reduce the rate of recurrence. Further analysis was conducted to identify the herbs that may be contributing to the effect seen in included clinical studies. There was some overlap in herbs in meta-analyses of clinical signs, patient-reported symptoms and recurrence (Table 5.27). *Fu ling* 茯苓 and *sheng di huang* 生地黄 appeared in frequently used herb lists for all three outcome categories.

Table 5.27. Frequently Reported Orally and Topically Used Herbs in Meta-analyses Showing Favourable Effect

Herbs	Scientific Name	Frequency of Use
Clinical signs: 1 meta-analysis, 5 RCTs.		
Long gu 龙骨	Fossilised bone	5
Duan mu li 煅牡蛎	*Ostrea* spp	4
Fu ling 茯苓	*Poria cocos* (Schw.) Wolf	3
Gu sui bu 骨碎补	*Drynaria fortunei* (Kunze) J. Sm.	3
Sheng di huang 生地黄	*Rehmannia glutinosa* Libosch.	3
Di fu zi 地肤子	*Kochia scoparia* (L.) Schrad.	2
Patient-reported symptoms: 1 meta-analysis, 4 RCTs.		
Sheng di huang 生地黄	*Rehmannia glutinosa* Libosch.	4
Dang gui 当归	*Angelica sinensis* (Oliv.) Diels	3
Fu ling 茯苓	*Poria cocos* (Schw.) Wolf	3
Bai xian pi 白鲜皮	*Dictamnus dasycarpus* Turcz.	2
Bai zhu 白术	*Atractylodes macrocephala* Koidz.	2
Recurrence: 1 meta-analysis, 3 RCTs.		
Gan cao 甘草	*Glycyrrhiza* spp	4
Sheng di huang 生地黄	*Rehmannia glutinosa* Libosch.	3
Long gu 龙骨	Fossilised bone	3
Bai zhu 白术	*Atractylodes macrocephala* Koidz.	2
Di fu zi 地肤子	*Kochia scoparia* (L.) Schrad.	2
Duan mu li 煅牡蛎	*Ostrea* spp	2
Fu ling 茯苓	*Poria cocos* (Schw.) Wolf	2
Gu sui bu 骨碎补	*Drynaria fortunei* (Kunze) J. Sm.	2
Huang bai 黄柏	*Phellodendron chinense* Schneid.	2
Huang lian 黄连	*Coptis* spp	2

Abbreviations: RCTs, randomised controlled trials.

Clinical signs: See 'SCOring of Atopic Dermatitis Index'. Patient-reported symptoms: See Table 5.26. Recurrence: See 'Recurrence'.

Note: 1) The frequency of use may be greater than the number of studies in the meta-analyses, as some studies included multiple CHM formulae; 2) The use of some herbs may be restricted in some countries. Readers are advised to comply with relevant regulations.

Both these herbs were also found in the top five herbs used in all oral plus topical CHM RCTs (see Table 5.23), so it is likely that the herbs used in studies included in favourable meta-analyses are indicative of the herbs used for research and clinical management of atopic dermatitis.

Safety of Oral plus Topical Chinese Herbal Medicine in Randomised Controlled Trials

Fourteen studies (H20, H51, H132–H135, H137–H140, H143, H145–H147) (652 participants in intervention groups and 630 in comparator groups) reported on adverse events. Four studies (H138–H140, H147) reported that no adverse events occurred during the trial. Studies which reported the occurrence of adverse events all compared oral plus topical CHM alone with pharmacotherapy or pharmacotherapy plus placebo. The number of adverse events with oral plus topical CHM was similar to that seen with pharmacotherapy (54 events vs. 49 events, respectively). Adverse events in the CHM groups were mostly gastrointestinal, including 35 cases of gastrointestinal discomfort/reactions and four cases of abdominal pain/diarrhoea. Other adverse events in the treatment groups included nine cases of common cold, four cases of mild headache, one case of elevated alanine aminotransferase which returned to normal after ceasing CHM and one unspecified adverse reaction. The types of adverse events in people who received pharmacotherapy varied. Adverse events included 18 cases of diarrhoea, nine cases of lethargy/fatigue, six cases of common cold, three cases of drowsiness, three cases of mild gastrointestinal reactions, two cases of skin pigmentation and atrophy, two cases of skin itch, burning and redness, six unspecified adverse reactions, and an unspecified number of cases of somnolence.

Controlled Clinical Trials of Oral plus Topical Chinese Herbal Medicine

One study (H148) evaluated the combination of oral plus topical CHM for atopic dermatitis. The study was conducted in China and included 60 participants. There were slightly more females than males (33 females compared to 27 males), and participant age ranged from 11 to 30 years. Chinese medicine syndromes which were used as inclusion criteria, were also used to guide treatment, and included wind-dampness encumbering the skin and Blood deficiency with wind-dryness. The study compared an investigator-developed formula for oral and topical use with TCS.

The study evaluated physician-assessed signs of atopic dermatitis using the SCORAD,[9] itch severity and recurrence. The combination of oral and topical CHM did not reduce the severity of atopic dermatitis signs on the SCORAD (60 participants, MD: –0.18 points [–5.94, 5.58]), or itch severity (60 participants, MD: –0.92 [–3.00, 1.16]). Furthermore, no difference between groups was seen in the rate of recurrence for all participants six months after treatment finished (57 participants, RR: 0.41 [0.09, 1.96]). The study did not report on adverse events.

Non-controlled Studies of Oral Plus Topical Chinese Herbal Medicine

The combination of oral and topical CHM was evaluated in 14 non-controlled studies (H149–H162), with 688 people participating in these studies. Two studies (H153, H160) were case reports, and the remaining 12 were case series. Studies used CM syndromes as an inclusion criterion and to guide treatment. Syndromes used as inclusion criteria included damp-heat syndrome (H153, H155), Blood heat and Blood dryness syndrome (H155), Kidney deficiency syndrome (H155), Spleen dampness syndrome (H153), Spleen deficiency and Blood dryness syndrome (H151), Spleen deficiency syndrome (H155), Liver depression syndrome (H155), and *yin* injury syndrome (H153). One syndrome that was used to guide treatment was reported in two studies (H154, H158): Blood deficiency with wind-dryness syndrome. Other syndromes included accumulation of damp-heat in the intestines (H160), Blood dryness (H155), Blood heat with Blood dryness (H155), Blood heat with wind-dryness (H154), damp-heat (H155), foetal Heat (H159), foetal toxicity and damp-heat syndrome (H154), fire toxin on the skin (H160), invasion of wind-heat transforming to damp heat with fire toxin on the skin (H160), Kidney deficiency (H155), Liver depression (H155), Spleen deficiency damp-heat (H158), Spleen deficiency (H155), *yin* deficiency (H159) and *yin* injury (H153).

Two studies (H153, H156) combined oral plus topical CHM with conventional medicine. Much like non-controlled studies of oral CHM, studies of oral plus topical CHM were primarily evaluating investigator-developed formulas. One oral CHM formula was used in two studies — *Dang gui yin zi* 当归饮子. There was no overlap in other oral CHM formulas, nor in formulas for topical application.

As this group of non-controlled studies evaluated both oral and topical CHM, the frequency of use of some herbs was greater than the number of studies. Not surprisingly, the most frequently used herbs in non-controlled studies evaluating oral plus topical CHM included herbs frequently used in oral CHM studies and those in topical CHM studies. *Gan cao* 甘草 was the most frequently used herb (20 uses), with other forms of *Glycyrrhiza* species, such as *sheng gan cao* 生甘草, also contributing to its high frequency (Table 5.28). Other frequently reported herbs included *ku shen* 苦参 (16 uses), *huang qin* 黄芩 (13 uses), *sheng di* 生地 (13 uses) and *dang gui* 当归 (12 uses).

Table 5.28. Frequently Reported Orally and Topically Used Herbs in Non-controlled Studies

Most Common Herbs	Scientific Name	Frequency of Use
Gan cao 甘草	*Glycyrrhiza* spp	20
Ku shen 苦参	*Sophora flavescens* Ait.	16
Huang qin 黄芩	*Scutellaria baicalensis* Georgi	13
Sheng di 生地	*Rehmannia glutinosa* Libosch.	13
Dang gui 当归	*Angelica sinensis* (Oliv.) Diels	12
Da qing ye 大青叶	*Isatis indigotica* Fort.	7
Dan shen 丹参	*Salvia miltiorrhiza* Bge.	7
Hu zhang 虎杖	*Polygonum cuspidatum* Sieb. et Zucc.	7
Mu dan pi 牡丹皮	*Paeonia suffruticosa* Andr.	7
Ye ju hua 野菊花	*Chrysanthemum indicum* L.	7
Bai ji li 白蒺藜	*Tribulus terrestris* L.	6
Bai xian pi 白鲜皮	*Dictamnus dasycarpus* Turcz.	6
Huang lian 黄连	*Coptis* spp	6
Jing jie 荆芥	*Schizonepeta tenuifolia* Briq.	6
Bing pian 冰片	Borneol	5
Chi shao 赤芍	*Paeonia* spp	5
Hua shi 滑石 *(liu yi san* 六一散)	Hydrated magnesium silicate	5 (1)
Huang qi 黄芪	*Astragalus* spp	5
Tu fu ling 土茯苓	*Smilax glabra* Roxb.	5

Note: The use of some herbs may be restricted in some countries. Readers are advised to comply with relevant regulations.

Safety of Oral plus Topical Chinese Herbal Medicine in Non-controlled Studies

Six studies involving 274 participants (H151, H152, H155, H156, H160, H161) reported on adverse events, with one study (H151) reporting no adverse events. Adverse events included gastrointestinal and dermatological events. Thirteen cases of diarrhoea were reported, as were two cases of contact dermatitis, one case of bloating and flatulence, and an unspecified number of cases of gastrointestinal discomfort.

Clinical Evidence for Commonly Used Chinese Herbal Medicine Treatments

Many of the formulas recommended in clinical guidelines and textbooks in Chapter 2 have been evaluated in clinical studies. The most frequently evaluated formula across all clinical studies was *Xiao feng san* 消风散, used in eight studies. Four RCTs (H5, H14, H21, H47) used *Xiao feng san* 消风散 alone as the intervention, and four non-controlled studies described *Xiao feng san* 消风散 along with other CHM formulas. Review of the evidence from RCTs was limited to studies where *Xiao feng san* 消风散 was evaluated alone, due to the difficulties in teasing out effects when multiple formulas are combined. When modified *Xiao feng san* 消风散 was compared with loratadine, the score on EASI[12] was significantly lower among participants who received CHM (80 participants, MD: −1.30 points [−1.48, −1.12], H5). A second study (H14) reported results using SASSAD;[13] however, data were not able to be re-analysed. The study reported that no adverse events were noted. *Xiao feng san* 消风散 was compared with placebo in one study (H47), although data were not presented in a way that allowed for further analysis. The authors described improvements in clinical lesions, erythema, skin surface damage, pruritus and sleep. Two cases of transient gastrointestinal upsets were reported in people who received *Xiao feng san* 消风散, and one case of transient increase in aspartate aminotransferase occurred, but group allocation was not described for this adverse event. One study (H21) used *Xiao feng san* 消风散 as an IM with loratadine and laser phototherapy. Data for SASSAD were not able to be analysed, and the study reported no adverse events.

Dang gui yin zi 当归饮子加减 was the second most frequently evaluated formula among those included in Chapter 2. *Dang gui yin zi* 当归饮子 was used in seven studies. Three RCTs (H32, H39, H142) described using *Dang gui yin zi* 当归饮子 and other CHM formulas, and one RCT (H23) used *Dang gui yin zi* 当归饮子 as an IM. Among the three non-controlled studies (H76, H154, H159), all described using *Dang gui yin zi* 当归饮子 with other CHM treatments. RCT evidence was available from one study (H23) for *Dang gui yin zi* 当归饮子加减 as an IM. When used in combination with TCS and loratadine, *Dang gui yin zi* 当归饮子加减 increased the chance of achieving 30%, or greater, improvement in signs and symptoms (80 participants, RR: 1.69 [1.13, 2.51]). No adverse events occurred during the trial.

The oral formula *Pei tu qing xin tang* 培土清心汤 was evaluated in one RCT (H51) and four non-controlled studies (H65, H69, H71, H72). All five studies used *Pei tu qing xin tang* 培土清心汤 alone as the intervention. Evidence from the RCT was not able to be re-analysed. The authors of this study concluded that *Pei tu qing xin tang* 培土清心汤 produced a significantly greater decrease in SCORAD[9] at weeks 28 and 36, a significantly greater change in patient self-assessment at 20 weeks through to the completion of follow-up, and a greater change in HRQoL on the DLQI[14]/CDLQI[15] at week 12, compared to the control group.

Other formulas described in Chapter 2 were evaluated less frequently. *Huang lian* ointment 黄连膏 was used in combination with other oral or topical CHMs in two studies: one RCT (H133) and one non-controlled study (H154). Similarly, *Gan cao* oil 甘草油 was used in combination with other CHM treatments in one RCT (H145) and one non-controlled study (H151). Six formulas described in Chapter 2 were evaluated in one clinical study:

- Modified *Qi pi wan* granules 加味启脾丸颗粒剂 were used alone as the intervention in one RCT (H15).
- *Qing dai* ointment 青黛油膏 was used with other oral and topical CHM formulas in one RCT (H143).

- *Run zao zhi yang jiao nang* 润燥止痒胶囊 was used with other oral CHM formulas in one case series (H66).
- *San xin dao chi san* 三心导赤散 was used in combination with other oral CHM formulas in one case series (H159).
- *Shen ling bai zhu san* 参苓白术散 was used in combination with other oral CHM formulas in one RCT (H32).
- *Xiao er hua shi tang* 小儿化湿汤 was used alone in one case series (H79).

Of the six formulas listed above, controlled trial evidence was able to be evaluated for one formula: modified *Qi pi wan* granules 加味启脾丸颗粒剂. Compared with cyproheptadine, modified *Qi pi wan* granules 加味启脾丸颗粒剂 were as effective at increasing the chance of 30%, or greater, improvement in signs and symptoms (51 participants, RR: 1.41 [0.88, 2.25], H15). No adverse events were reported in the CHM group.

In summary, many of the CHM formulas described in Chapter 2 have been evaluated in clinical studies. Researchers have frequently combined these formulas with other oral or topical CHM formulas. While this may be reflective of clinical practice, it prevents further analysis of the efficacy of individual formulas. Evidence from single studies suggests *Xiao feng san* 消风散 may reduce score on EASI[12] and *Dang gui yin zi* 当归饮子加减 may improve signs and symptoms. Further evidence is needed to confirm these findings.

Summary of Chinese Herbal Medicine Clinical Evidence

The evidence for CHM in atopic dermatitis is growing. This chapter has reviewed the clinical evidence for studies that met the inclusion criteria described in Chapter 4, but many other studies evaluating CHM exist that have not been critically evaluated here. The number of RCTs outweighed the number of CCTs and non-controlled studies, suggesting a focus on generating high-level clinical evidence. Oral CHM was evaluated more frequently than topical CHM, or the combination of oral and topical CHM. Treatments tended to be of short duration, ranging from seven days to 24 weeks. The median treatment frequency in RCTs was four weeks. When follow-up assessment was conducted, this usually took place within six months of the end of treatment. More studies with longer duration of treatment and follow-up assessment are needed in order to provide evidence for the potential role of CHM in the long-term management of atopic dermatitis.

Almost one-third of studies (51 of the 163 included studies) used syndrome differentiation as an inclusion criterion and/or to guide treatment. Three CM syndromes from clinical guidelines and textbooks in Chapter 2 were described in CHM clinical studies: wind-dampness encumbering the skin, Spleen deficiency with dampness retention and Blood deficiency with wind-dryness. While not directly matching the syndromes in Chapter 2, many of the key concepts were also captured in clinical studies. For example, syndromes of damp-heat or wind-damp-heat were described in clinical studies. The concepts of wind, damp and heat are all presented in syndromes in Chapter 2. The similarity in syndromes suggests that clinical studies were evaluating syndromes relevant to atopic dermatitis.

Many of the included studies evaluated formulas developed by study investigators. It was not always clear whether a formula was a modification of an existing formula that had been renamed. As frequency analysis was conducted based on formula name, it is possible that the actual number of formulas investigated may be less than calculated, and the frequency for some traditional formulas may be higher than reported.

Two oral CHM formulas, *Xiao feng san* 消风散 and *Dang gui yin zi* 当归饮子, were among those used in multiple clinical studies (eight and seven, respectively). These two formulas are recommended in the key clinical textbooks and guidelines included in Chapter 2, and were found in classical literature citations in Chapter 3. These oral formulas may be promising treatments, although it was not possible to conduct GRADE assessment of the quality of the evidence for these treatments. *Fu fang gan cao suan gan pian* (compound glycyrrhizin tablets) 复方甘草酸苷片 was evaluated in six clinical studies, four of which were RCTs. Due to differences in comparators and outcomes, data were not able to be pooled for analysis. The efficacy of this manufactured product remains unclear. Few topical CHM treatments were evaluated in multiple clinical studies, with *huang lian* ointment 黄连软膏 and *jin huang* cream 金黄膏 being used in two studies each. While *huang lian* ointment 黄连软膏 has been recommended in the clinical textbooks and guidelines described in Chapter 2, *jin huang* cream 金黄膏 has not. This formula was used in two studies by the same investigator, so the fact that it has been used in multiple studies does not equate to common clinical usage.

The majority of controlled trials compared CHMs with guideline-recommended treatments. Few studies compared CHM with placebo or no treatment. In studies that compared CHM with pharmacotherapy, antihistamines were the most frequently used comparator. Oral antihistamines are recommended in some international guidelines as adjunctive therapy[19,20] and/or for the management of pruritus.[21] Fewer studies compared CHM with emollients, TCS or TCIs, despite their use as first-line therapy.

Clinician-assessed signs and patient-reported symptoms were most commonly evaluated in controlled trials. Clinician-assessed signs were most commonly evaluated using SCORAD[9] and EASI,[12] while patient-reported symptoms related to pruritus and sleep disturbance. Results from meta-analyses of RCTs found that oral CHM used alone, or as an IM, improved outcomes on SCORAD, as did topical CHM as an IM and oral plus topical CHM used alone. Oral CHM as an IM reduced the severity of itch and sleep disturbance, compared with pharmacotherapy, and the combination of oral plus topical CHM reduced itch severity. These results indicate a potential role for CHM in improving sign and symptom severity.

An interesting finding was a reduction in SCORAD, indicating better clinical outcomes, when oral CHM was compared with pharmacotherapy alone. All studies included in this analysis used antihistamines as the pharmacotherapy comparator. Subjective symptoms, including pruritus and sleep loss, is one of the three components of SCORAD, with the other two being the extent of disease and severity of erythema, oedema/papulation, oozing/crusting, excoriation, and lichenification. While antihistamines may reduce pruritus, they are less likely to affect other clinical signs. Therefore, it is not surprising that oral CHM improved the signs and symptoms of atopic dermatitis more than a treatment that targets one symptom only.

The impact of atopic dermatitis on HRQoL was less frequently evaluated. Results were largely from single RCTs. Conflicting findings were seen with oral CHM, where one study found worse HRQoL compared to the antihistamine epinastine, and another found no difference when oral CHM was compared to pharmacotherapy plus placebo. One study found a lower mean score on the DLQI[14] with oral CHM as an IM. Similarly, conflicting results were also found from single studies of topical CHM, and the combination of oral and topical CHM. The evidence for CHM on HRQoL is limited.

In studies that reported measures of quality of life, several used age-appropriate outcome measures. For example, several studies used the DLQI[14] for adults and CDLQI[15] for children who participated in the study. When it came to reporting results, the results for both outcome measures were reported in aggregate. This approach has been criticised by the developers of these outcome measures, as each tool has questions specific for the age group in which the instrument is used.[22] Finlay and Basra (2012)[22] recommend that statistical analysis be conducted for each outcome measure separately. Studies included in this review did not report results of each outcome tool separately. Results that were presented in aggregate have been analysed and presented in the relevant sections above; however, findings should be interpreted in light of the recommendation from developers.

Long-term control is recognised as one of the core outcomes by the Harmonizing Outcome Measures for Eczema (HOME) group.[23] Consensus is yet to be reached on how long-term control should be measured. Systematic reviews have highlighted diversity in how long-term control is measured,[24] with differences in the definition of acute exacerbation and few studies measuring patient-reported flares.[25] Recent research has proposed the use of 'well-controlled weeks' for atopic dermatitis, a concept that has been used to assess long-term control for asthma.[26] Again, no consensus has been reached on the definition of a well-controlled week.

The majority of RCTs in this review measured the number of participants experiencing recurrence at a specified time point. Results from meta-analyses showed that oral CHM alone, or as an IM, reduced the chance of recurrence within six months. Topical CHM as an IM also reduced the chance of recurrence within six months. The combination of oral and topical CHM appeared to have longer term effects, with meta-analysis showing a reduced chance of recurrence six months, or longer, after the end of treatment.

Included studies infrequently provided definitions as to what constituted recurrence, nor were details provided about the method of assessments. For example, flares may be self-reported, or assessed at scheduled or unscheduled clinic visits. Differences were noted in the number of participants who were assessed; for example, some studies assessed all participants while others assessed only those judged to have a clinical cure at the end of treatment. Furthermore, the time point at which recurrence was assessed ranged from 'within four weeks' to one year. Pragmatic decisions were made in grouping studies according to who was assessed, and when follow-up assessment was made (less than six months, or six months or greater). It is possible that different decisions, in relation to analysis, would produce different results.

Chinese herbal medicine is not without side effects. Mild adverse events were reported in many studies, and often related to the route of administration. In orally administered CHM, gastrointestinal complaints such as nausea, diarrhoea and abdominal discomfort were more frequent. When CHM was applied topically, adverse events were dermatological in nature. Events included burning, itching or stinging sensations on the skin, and skin flushing. Patients should be advised of the possibility of such events and practitioners may consider modifications if adverse events are bothersome.

Several limitations were noted in the evidence. The methodological reporting of the quality of studies varied, and none were free from bias. Few studies blinded participants, personnel and outcome assessors to group allocation. When assessing patient-reported outcomes, the potential for bias needs to be considered. Details relating to assessment of outcomes were lacking, for example, timing of, and criteria for, assessment. Many of the studies were conducted in China and published in Chinese, suggesting publication bias may exist. Furthermore, it was clear that some studies evaluated the efficacy and safety of CHM for atopic dermatitis in children. This information was not reported in other studies and the decision was made to pool studies where possible regardless of participant age. The findings described may not apply for different subpopulations. Practitioners should use their clinical judgment when selecting treatments based on syndrome differentiation.

References

1. Armstrong NC, Ernst E. (1999) The treatment of eczema with Chinese herbs: A systematic review of randomized clinical trials. *Br J Clin Pharmacol* **48**(2): 262–264.

2. Gu S, Yang AW, Xue CC, *et al.* (2013) Chinese herbal medicine for atopic eczema. *The Cochrane Database of Systematic Reviews* **9**: CD008642.

3. Gu S, Yang AW, Li CG, *et al.* (2014) Topical application of Chinese herbal medicine for atopic eczema: A systematic review with a meta-analysis. *Dermatology* **228**(4): 294–302.

4. Shi ZF, Song TB, Xie J, *et al.* (2017) The traditional Chinese medicine and relevant treatment for the efficacy and safety of atopic dermatitis: A systematic review and meta-analysis of randomized controlled trials. *Evid Based Complement Alternat Med* **2017**: 6026434.

5. Tan HY, Zhang AL, Chen D, *et al.* (2013) Chinese herbal medicine for atopic dermatitis: A systematic review. *J Am Acad Dermatol* **69**(2): 295–304.

6. 杨素清, 张鑫, 刘璐佳. (2016) 中药治疗特应性皮炎 meta 分析. 辽宁中医药大学学报 **18**(19): 9–12.

7. 龚小红. (2009) 中医药治疗异位性皮炎 meta 分析. 中华中医药学刊 **27**(07): 1425–1427.

8. 吴卿, 阮红石, 赵巍, 莫秀梅, 温晓文, 陈达灿. (2015) 中医外治法治疗特应性皮炎的 meta 分析 [j]. 中华中医药杂志 **30**(12): 4462–4465.

9. (1993) Severity scoring of atopic dermatitis: The SCORAD index. Consensus report of the European Task Force on Atopic Dermatitis. *Dermatology* **186**: 23–31.

10. 国家中医药管理局. (1994) 中医病证诊断疗效标准. 南京: 南京大学出版社.

11. 郑筱萸. (2002) 中药新药临床研究指导原则(试行). 北京: 中国医药科技出版社.

12. Tofte S, Graeber M, Cherill R, *et al.* (1998) Eczema area and severity index (EASI): A new tool to evaluate atopic dermatitis. *J Eur Acad Dermatol Venereol* **11**: S197.

13. Berth-Jones J. (1996) Six area, six sign atopic dermatitis (SASSAD) severity score: A simple system for monitoring disease activity in atopic dermatitis. *Br J Dermatol* **135**(Suppl 48): 25–30.

14. Finlay A, Khan G. (1994) Dermatology life quality index (DLQI): A simple practical measure for routine clinical use. *Clin Exp Dermatol* **19**(3): 210–216.

15. Lewis-Jones MS, Finlay AY. (1995) The Children's Dermatology Life Quality Index (CDLQI): Initial validation and practical use. *Br J Dermatol* **132**(6): 942–949.

16. Wolkerstorfer A, de Waard Van der Spek FB, Glazenburg EJ, *et al.* (1999) Scoring the severity of atopic dermatitis: Three item severity score as a rough system for daily practice and as a pre-screening tool for studies. *Acta Dermatol Venereol* **79**(5): 356–359.

17. Rajka G, Langeland T. (1989) Grading of the severity of atopic dermatitis. *Acta Dermatol Venereol Suppl* **144**: 13–14.

18. Lewis-Jones MS, Finlay AY, Dykes PJ. (2001) The Infants' Dermatitis Quality of Life Index. *Br J Dermatol* **144**(1): 104–110.

19. Katayama I, Aihara M, Ohya Y, *et al.* (2017) Japanese guidelines for atopic dermatitis 2017. *Allergol Int* **66**(2): 230–247.

20. Kim J, Kim H, Lew B, *et al.* (2015) Consensus guidelines for the treatment of atopic dermatitis in Korea (Part II): Systemic treatment. *Ann Dermatol* **27**(5): 578–592.

21. Rubel D, Thirumoorthy T, Soebaryo RW, *et al.* (2013) Consensus guidelines for the management of atopic dermatitis: An Asia-Pacific perspective. *J Dermatol* **40**(3): 160–171.

22. Finlay AY, Basra MK. (2012) DLQI and CDLQI scores should not be combined. *Br J Dermatol* **167**(2): 453–454.

23. Chalmers JR, Simpson E, Apfelbacher CJ, *et al.* (2016) Report from the fourth international consensus meeting to harmonize core outcome measures for atopic eczema/dermatitis clinical trials (HOME initiative). *Br J Dermatol* **175**(1): 69–79.

24. Barbarot S, Rogers NK, Abuabara K, *et al.* (2016) Strategies used for measuring long-term control in atopic dermatitis trials: A systematic review. *J Am Acad Dermatol* **75**(5): 1038–1044.

25. Langan SM, Schmitt J, Williams HC, *et al.* (2014) How are eczema 'flares' defined? A systematic review and recommendation for future studies. *Br J Dermatol.* **170**(3): 548–556.

26. Langan SM, Stuart B, Bradshaw L, *et al.* (2017) Measuring long-term disease control in patients with atopic dermatitis: A validation study of well-controlled weeks. *J Allergy Clin Immunol* **140**(6): 1580–1586.

References for Included Chinese Herbal Medicine Clinical Studies

Study No.	Reference
H1	陈保疆, 张玉环. (2011) 健脾利湿汤治疗异位性皮炎的疗效观察与相关实验研究. 吉林中医药 **31**(4): 335–336.
H2	陈海兵. (2014) 复方甘草酸苷片联合氯雷他定分散片治疗特应性皮炎的临床治疗效果观察. 中国医疗美容 **5**: 108.
H3	陈佳. (2011) 双黄汤治疗小儿特应性皮炎临床观察. 成都: 成都中医药大学.
H4	董心亚, 周健. (2015) 健脾化湿汤联合丁酸氢化可的松乳膏治疗特应性皮炎的效果. 广东医学 **36**(22): 3540–3542.
H5	傅佩骏. (2013) 消风散治疗特应性皮炎的疗效观察. 中成药 **35**(12): 2762–2763.
H6	胡永顺, 张宝霞 郭玉平. (2013) 中西医结合治疗特应性皮炎的随机对照研究. 中医临床研究 **5**(3): 10–12.
H7	黄咏菁, 陈达灿, 莫秀梅. (2004) 健脾渗湿冲剂治疗儿童异位性皮炎脾虚证的临床观察. 陕西中医 **25**(5): 396–398.
H8	金培志, 叶秋华, 沈明. (2007) 健脾止痒颗粒治疗特应性皮炎 32 例疗效观察. 河南中医 **27**(12): 61–62.
H9	瞿平元, 蔡正良, 李亚琴, *et al.* (2010) 清热祛风汤治疗特应性皮炎 30 例临床疗效观察. 甘肃医药 **29**(6): 646–648.
H10	李勇, 廖梦怡, 李东海, *et al.* (2011) 健脾养阴法治疗特应性皮炎临床研究. 新中医. **43**(2): 92–93.
H11	林海桂. (2006) 健脾利湿汤治疗儿童异位性皮炎 136 例.浙江中医杂志 **41**(7): 392.

(Continued)

(*Continued*)

Study No.	Reference
H12	刘源, 叶秋华, 陈加媛, *et al.* (2007) 中西医结合治疗儿童特应性皮炎临床研究. 南京中医药大学学报. **23**(2): 93–95.
H13	吕慧青, 华红, 郑玮清, *et al.* (2016) 加味滋阴除湿汤治疗小儿特应性皮炎疗效观察及对 SCORAD 评分与血清总 IgE 的影响. 现代中医临床. **23**(6): 36–38.
H14	罗凤娇. (2010) 消风散加减治疗异位性皮炎之疗效评估. 南京中医药大学.
H15	麻林玖, 梁红梅. (2006) 加味启脾丸颗粒治疗儿童特应性皮炎疗效观察. 中国皮肤性病学杂志 **20**(11): 698.
H16	毛群先, 蓝善辉, 余土根. (2008) 辨证论治联合综合护理治疗特应性皮炎的临床观察. 护理研究 **14**: 1276–1277.
H17	倪文琼, 定巍, 于江东, *et al.* (2000) 三组药物治疗异位性皮炎前后血清 IL-4 和总 IgE 的临床研究. 河南诊断与治疗杂志. **14**(3): 174–175.
H18	欧柏生, 刘卫兵, 王建民. (2006) 四弯风汤联合西药治疗特应性皮炎 34 例. 中国民间疗法 **14**(1): 8–9.
H19	彭勇, 李斌, 李锋, *et al.* (2013) 健脾祛风方治疗特应性皮炎 95 例临床观察. 上海中医药大学学报 **27**(3): 45–47.
H20	饶美荣. (2010) 清心培土法治疗特应性皮炎的临床研究. 南京: 南京中医药大学.
H21	佘虹丽. (2011) 消风散对特应性皮炎患者的临床疗效及尘螨变应原的影响. 南宁: 广西中医药大学.
H22	石婧, 刁友涛, 李晓伟. (2012) 复方中药治疗特应性皮炎疗效及对免疫功能调节作用研究. 中国中西医结合皮肤性病学杂志 **11**(3): 143–145.
H23	史永俭, 张春敏, 马冬梅, *et al.* (2008) 中西医结合治疗特应性皮炎的临床观察. 中国中西医结合杂志 **28**(8): 686–688.
H24	宋飞妮. (2015) 健脾养血汤治疗特应性皮炎临床观察. 深圳中西医结合杂志. **25**(22): 51–52.
H25	孙晓冬. (2006) 健脾渗湿颗粒治疗特应性皮炎的疗效评价及其对复发的影响. 广州：广州中医药大学.
H26	孙岩, 余展国. (2011) 苦参片口服联合窄谱中波紫外线照射对特应性皮炎患者外周血嗜酸细胞影响的探讨. 贵阳中医学院学报 **33**(4): 75–77.
H27	王金玲. (2016)自拟地芍玄乌汤治疗异位性皮炎 45 例. 基层医学论坛 **20**(30): 4260–4261.
H28	王榴慧, 周莲宝. (2002) 清热利湿合剂治疗儿童过敏性湿疹 648 例临床观察. 上海中医药大学学报 **16**(1): 26–27.

(*Continued*)

(Continued)

Study No.	Reference
H29	巫毅, 李晓天, 杨凌伟, *et al.* (2008) 复方甘草酸苷联合左西替利嗪治疗儿童特应性皮炎疗效观察. 中国麻风皮肤病杂志 **24**(8): 660–661.
H30	吴蓓玲, 曹毅, 程立峰, *et al.* (2012) 皮炎消净饮 II 号联合窄谱中波紫外线对特应性皮炎患者细胞黏附分子及总 IgE 的影响. 中华中医药杂志 **27**(5): 1317–1320.
H31	吴香香, 胡瑞. (2015) 复方甘草酸苷片联合蓝润、地奈德乳膏治疗特应性皮炎疗效观察及生活质量评价. 医学信息 **28**(28): 109–110.
H32	吴允波, 邱桂荣, 许来宾. (2014) 中医辨证联合开瑞坦治疗特应性皮炎 43 例临床观察. 江苏中医药 **46**(6): 49–50.
H33	徐岳清, 陈新. (2016) 健脾化湿汤联合丁酸氢化可的松乳膏治疗特应性皮炎的疗效分析. 大家健康 (下旬版) **10**(27): 28–29.
H34	薛素琴, 谭金华. (2011) 生血润肤饮加减治疗儿童特应性皮炎临床观察. 新中医 **43**(2): 94–95.
H35	杨爱荣, 彭关连, 余霞萍, *et al.* (2013) 消异止痒汤加减治疗儿童期特应性皮炎 45 例. 中国实验方剂学杂志 **25**(4): 309–311.
H36	杨雪松, 叶建州, 李钦. (2009) 健脾养血祛风法治疗特应性皮炎临床疗效及对皮肤屏障功能的影响. 云南中医学院学报 **32**(3): 5–7.
H37	叶挺挺. (2014) 76 例特应性皮炎中医辨证论治对照疗效观察. 中国地方病防治杂志 **29**(2): 417.
H38	张池金. (2011) 滋阴清热法治疗特应性皮炎 30 例临床观察. 中医药导报 **17**(8): 22–24.
H39	张娟. (2012) 中医药治疗异位性皮炎临床研究. 中医学报 **27**(7): 897–898.
H40	张彤. (2013) 四虫消风散治疗儿童重症特应性皮炎 60 例临床观察. 中国社区医师 **15**(7): 192.
H41	张葳. (2014) 加味滋阴除湿汤治疗特应性皮炎的临床观察. 黑龙江: 黑龙江中医药大学.
H42	郑义辉. (2014) 复方甘草酸苷片联合氯雷他定分散片治疗特应性皮炎的疗效分析. 当代医学 **20**(17): 126–127.
H43	周琳. (2012) 滋阴健脾冲剂治疗特应性皮炎的疗效观察. 武汉:湖北中医药大学.
H44	周增民. (2016) 祛风四物汤结合氯雷他定治疗特应性皮炎临床观察. 中国中医药科技 **23**(1): 93–94.
H45	周智敏. (2003) 中西医结合治疗异位性皮炎 41 例临床研究. 湖南中医药导报 **9**(3): 34–35.

(Continued)

(Continued)

Study No.	Reference
H46	朱春友. (2001) 中西医结合治疗异位性皮炎疗效观察. 现代医药卫生 **17**(5): 368.
H47	Cheng HM, Chiang LC, Jan YM, *et al.* (2011) The efficacy and safety of a Chinese herbal product (Xiao-Feng-San) for the treatment of refractory atopic dermatitis: A randomized, double-blind, placebo-controlled trial. *Int Arch Allergy Immunol* **155**(2): 141–148.
H48	Fung AY, Look PC, Chong LY, *et al.* (1999) A controlled trial of traditional Chinese herbal medicine in Chinese patients with recalcitrant atopic dermatitis. *Int J Dermatol* **38**(5): 387–392.
H49	Hon KL, Leung TF, Ng PC, *et al.* (2007) Efficacy and tolerability of a Chinese herbal medicine concoction for treatment of atopic dermatitis: A randomized, double-blind, placebo-controlled study. *Br J Dermatol* **157**(2): 357–363.
H50	Kobayashi H, Ishii M, Takeuchi S, *et al.* (2010) Efficacy and safety of a traditional herbal medicine, hochu-ekki-to, in the long-term management of kikyo (delicate constitution) patients with atopic dermatitis: A 6-month, multicenter, double-blind, randomized, placebo-controlled study. *Evid Based Complement Alternat Med* **7**(3): 367–373.
H51	Liu J, Mo X, Wu D, *et al.* (2015) Efficacy of a Chinese herbal medicine for the treatment of atopic dermatitis: A randomised controlled study. *Complement Ther Med* **23**(5): 644–651.
H52	鲍丽霞. (2009) 自拟润肤止痒汤配合西药治疗特应性皮炎 37 例疗效观察. 中国中医药科技 **16**(3): 177.
H53	陈海亭, 赵晔, 巴东霞, *et al.* (2003) 丹参酮联合氢化可的松乳膏治疗特应性皮炎疗效观察. 临床皮肤科杂志 **32**(2): 110.
H54	陈艺明, 林金宝, 黄海松, *et al.* (2006) 滋阴熄风汤治疗特应性皮炎临床疗效观察. 临床皮肤科杂志 **35**(1): 55–56.
H55	李雪娇. (2011) 特异性免疫治疗联合玉屏风颗粒治疗特应性皮炎的疗效观察. 山东大学学报 (医学版) **49**(7): 144–146.
H56	张卫华, 徐霞, 任敏. (2011) 复方甘草酸苷联合盐酸非索非那定治疗儿童特应性皮炎疗效观察. 中国中西医结合皮肤性病学杂志 **10**(5): 312–313.
H57	邹继承. (2015) 健脾止痒汤治疗特应性皮炎的效果探析. 中国继续医学教育 **7**(22): 166–167.
H58	车武. (2015) 温清饮治疗异位性皮炎的临床回顾性总结. 北京: 北京中医药大学.

(Continued)

(Continued)

Study No.	Reference
H59	车武. (2005) 四虫止痒汤治疗成人异位性皮炎 62 例. 承德医学院学报 **22**(1): 38–39.
H60	陈妙善. (2003) 健脾运湿法治疗异位性湿疹 45 例. 江苏中医药 **24**(9): 39.
H61	陈伟斌. (2007) 清热活血祛风法治疗异位性皮炎体会. 云南中医中药杂志 **28**(3): 23–24.
H62	董子亮. (1997) 陈木森,菊池,顺一郎,奇妙饮治疗遗传过敏性皮炎临床观察. 中国中医药信息杂志 **4**(12): 36–37.
H63	宫崎纯, 杜金行, 史载祥. (1995) 中医药治愈异位性皮炎2例. 中日友好医院学报 **9**(4): 194.
H64	贯剑, 郑湘瑞, 何裕民, *et al.* (2006) 敏康片调整青少年过敏体质的临床研究. 北京中医药大学学报 **29**(8): 566–568.
H65	黄业坚. (2010) 清心培土法治疗特应性皮炎的疗效及对患者免疫调节作用的研究. 广州: 广州中医药大学.
H66	蒋靖. (2009) 润燥止痒胶囊联合荆防冲剂治疗特应性皮炎临床观察. 中国中西医结合皮肤性病学杂志 **8**(6): 376.
H67	孔兢谊, 任润媛, 刘晚霞. (2014) 麻杏石甘汤加味治疗皮肤病验案举隅. 现代中医药 **34**(6): 23–24.
H68	李晰, 李凛, 李树元. (2008) 四妙丸临床应用举隅. 中国中医药现代远程教育 **6**(1): 50.
H69	廖勇梅, 黎昌强, 陈德宇, *et al.* (2012) 培土清心方治疗特应性皮炎的疗效观察及对血清 NGF, SP 影响的研究. 辽宁中医杂志 **39**(12): 2344–2346.
H70	林珠. (1996) 清热利湿法治疗异位性皮炎 36 例. 北京中医 (4): 34–35.
H71	刘炽. (2009) 清心培土法对特应性皮炎患者 IL-2/TNF-α 及其受体的影响和疗效评价. 广州: 广州中医药大学.
H72	刘俊峰. (2010) 培土清心方对特应性皮炎患者血清 n-6 EFAs 及行为的影响. 广州: 广州中医药大学.
H73	沈昱颖, 沈华军. (2009) 犀角地黄汤加味治疗特应性皮炎 60 例. 山东中医杂志 **28**(6): 399.
H74	石汉振, 曾冬玉, 陈达灿, *et al.* (2011) 健脾渗湿法治疗特应性皮炎患者血清总 IgE, IgG, IgG4 变化及疗效评价. 中国中西医结合皮肤性病学杂志 **10**(1): 20–22.
H75	万英, 赵相雨. (2016) 辨证论治小儿特应性皮炎. 光明中医 **31**(9): 1311–1313.
H76	王琳. (2003) 90 例异位性皮炎的临床研究. 中国中西医结合皮肤性病学杂志 **2**(1): 46–47.

(Continued)

(*Continued*)

Study No.	Reference
H77	王欣. (2006) 健脾渗湿法治疗特应性皮炎的疗效及对患者免疫功能调节作用的研究. 广州: 广州中医药大学.
H78	王雄, 郎娜, 付中学. (2017) 黄尧洲教授从心论治特应性皮炎经验介绍. 世界中西医结合杂志 **12**(1): 40–42.
H79	魏跃钢, 单敏. (1993) 小儿化湿汤加减治疗小儿异位性皮炎 42 例. 南京中医学院学报 **9**(3): 52.
H80	吴蓓玲, 杨晓红, 曹毅, *et al.* (2012) 皮炎消净饮 II 号联合窄谱 UVB 照射治疗血虚风燥型特应性皮炎的临床及免疫组化研究. 中华中医药学刊 **30**(3): 559–561.
H81	杨晓红, 杨晓红, 代群, *et al.* (2013) 皮炎消净饮 I 号治疗特应性皮炎的临床及实验研究. 中国麻风皮肤病杂志 **29**(5): 334.
H82	曾少山. (2015) 异位性皮炎的中医证治研究. 南京: 南京中医药大学.
H83	张晓春. (2007) 运用中医卫气营血辨证治疗变态反应性皮肤病 258 例疗效分析. 湖南中医杂志 **23**(6): 23–25.
H84	张肖琴, 陈健民. (2015) 陈健民教授采用麻杏苡甘汤治疗儿童特应性皮炎临证经验. 亚太传统医药 **11**(23): 76–77.
H85	张玉环, 陈保疆, 杨慧文. (2004) 雷公藤多甙治疗异位性皮炎的临床观察. 中华现代中西医杂志 **2**(7): 131–132.
H86	郑继达, 刘广台. (1996) 中西医结合治疗异位性皮炎 36 例. 广西中医药 **19**(2): 15–16.
H87	周海啸. (2000) 中医辨证治疗异位性皮炎临床观察. 中国中医药信息杂志 **7**(10): 52–53.
H88	朱海莉. (2009) CDLQI、DFI 的译制与考评及对清心培土法治疗特应性皮炎患者的测评. 广州中医药大学.
H89	朱雨生. (1996) 青龙肠溶胶囊治疗儿童顽固性皮肤病 79 例疗效观察. 蛇志 **6**(1): 54–56.
H90	Atherton D, Sheehan M, Rustin MH, *et al.* (1990) Chinese herbs for eczema. *Lancet* **336**(8725): 1254.
H91	Hon KL, Leung TF, Wong Y, *et al.* (2004) A pentaherbs capsule as a treatment option for atopic dermatitis in children: An open-labeled case series. *Am J Chin Med* **32**(6): 941–950.
H92	Hon KL, Lo W, Cheng WK, *et al.* (2012) Prospective self-controlled trial of the efficacy and tolerability of a herbal syrup for young children with eczema. *J Dermatolog Treat* **23**(2): 116–121.

(*Continued*)

(Continued)

Study No.	Reference
H93	Kalus U, Pruss A, Bystron J, *et al.* (2003) Effect of Nigella sativa (black seed) on subjective feeling in patients with allergic diseases. *Phytother Res* **17**(10): 1209–1214.
H94	陈建宏, 范瑞强, 陈修漾, *et al.* (2012) 浅谈自拟金鱼外洗方对儿童异位性湿疹皮损严重程度的影响. 求医问药 (下半月) **10**(5): 319–320.
H95	陈建宏, 何秀玉. (2017) 金鱼外洗方对不同中医体质小儿异位性皮炎的疗效观察. 广州中医药大学学报 **34**(1): 35–39.
H96	陈建宏, 潘佩光, 范瑞强, *et al.* (2012) 金鱼外洗方治疗儿童湿热型异位性湿疹临床研究. 新中医 **44**(8): 113–115.
H97	陈建宏, 萧敏英, 杨敏莲. (2016) 金鱼外洗方外用治疗儿童异位性皮炎患儿疗效观察. 按摩与康复医学 **7**(21): 33–35.
H98	龚小俊. (2016) 三味清热止痒洗剂联合糖皮质激素治疗特应性皮炎疗效观察. 医学临床研究 **33**(9): 1712–1715.
H99	关健缨, 郑永平, 马立坚, *et al.* (2009) 消炎止痒洗剂治疗异位性皮炎的临床观察. 中国中医药现代远程教育 **7**(7): 138–139.
H100	郭樱. (2015) 复方榴莲皮软膏治疗特应性皮炎的疗效观察. 广州: 广州中医药大学.
H101	郭游, 叶建州. (2011) 外用润肤止痒散治疗特应性皮炎的临床观察. 皮肤病与性病 **33**(2): 100–101.
H102	黄晶, 杨玉峰, 陈宝清, *et al.* (2016) 复方榴莲皮软膏对 120 例特应性皮炎皮肤屏障功能修复的临床研究. 黑龙江中医药 **45**(2): 24–25.
H103	黄文晖, 王崇敏. (2016) 中药药浴联合他克莫司治疗儿童中、重度特应性皮炎的疗效及对血清 LTB_4, LTC_4 的影响. 中华全科医学 **14**(4): 604–606.
H104	刘慧焕, 李焕平. (2007) 中药煎剂联合糖皮质激素软膏治疗特应性皮炎疗效观察. 中国冶金工业医学杂志 **24**(5): 579–580.
H105	楼宏亮, 方国兴, 胡国华. (2015) 氯雷他定糖浆联合羌月乳膏治疗小儿特应性皮炎 65 例疗效观察. 中医儿科杂志 **11**(4): 42–43.
H106	罗维丹, 邬成霖. (2002) 复方苦参洗液治疗湿疹 60 例临床观察. 中国皮肤性病学杂志 **16**(2): 125–126.
H107	毛娟娟, 朱明芳, 张晓玲. (2014) 石榴皮软膏治疗特应性皮炎 30 例临床观察. 湖南中医杂志 **30**(4): 23–24.
H108	陶以成, 郎娜, 余远遥, *et al.* (2015) 金黄膏治疗特应性皮炎 45 例. 西部中医药 **28**(6): 100–101.

(Continued)

(*Continued*)

Study No.	Reference
H109	陶以成, 郎娜, 佘远遥, *et al.* (2014) 金黄膏对特应性皮炎患者血清肠毒素 B 及相关抗体的影响. 湖北中医杂志 **36**(9): 6–7.
H110	王海棠, 林素财, 郑永平, *et al.* (2015) 肤悦康洗剂对特应性皮炎患者 Th17, IL-17 的表达影响. 光明中医. **30**(9): 1904–1905.
H111	晏勇, 彭美连, 余霞萍, *et al.* (2013) 湿润烧伤膏治疗轻中度特应性皮炎的疗效观察. 中国烧伤创疡杂志 (4): 309–311.
H112	张怀镱, 霍晏, 罗静, *et al.* (2016) 肤舒止痒膏联合地奈德乳膏治疗儿童特应性皮炎的疗效观察. 转化医学电子杂志. **3**(5): 20–22.
H113	张晓燕, 杨丽芸, 杨丽君, *et al.* (2012) 七味解毒活血膏治疗小儿特应性皮炎的疗效分析. 中国美容医学 **21**(11): 225–226.
H114	张旭, 陈红旗. (2004) 丁香罗勒乳膏治疗异位性皮炎的临床研究. 中华实用中西医杂志 **4**(17): 3552–3554.
H115	张振榜, 刘胜. (2008) 冰黄肤乐软膏治疗成人特应性皮炎临床疗效观察. 四川中医 **26**(10): 95.
H116	Yen CY, Hsieh CL. (2016) Therapeutic effect of Tzu-yun ointment on patients with atopic dermatitis: A preliminary, randomized, controlled, open-label study. *J Altern Complement Med* **22**(3): 237–243.
H117	Saeedi M, Morteza-Semnani K, Ghoreishi MR. (2003) The treatment of atopic dermatitis with licorice gel. *J Dermatolog Treat* **14**(3): 153–157.
H118	杨丽君, 张晓燕, 李云霞, *et al.* (2012) 中药浴治疗小儿特应性皮炎 110 例疗效观察及中西医理论探讨. 中国美容医学 **21**(11): 215.
H119	张雪平. (2014) 中药外洗治疗婴儿湿疹. 内蒙古中医药 **17**: 23.
H120	简丹, 陈翔, 杜乾君, *et al.* (2009) 含马齿苋及牛油果树提取物护肤品辅助治疗特应性皮炎临床疗效观察. 临床皮肤科杂志 **38**(6): 367–369.
H121	Higaki S, Kitagawa T, Morohashi M, *et al.* (1999) Efficacy of Shiunko for the treatment of atopic dermatitis. *J Int Med Res* **27**(3): 143–147.
H122	程维芬, 邹学敏. (2008) 中药熏蒸加保湿润肤霜治疗特应性皮炎的护理. 中华现代护理学杂志 **5**(16): 1462–1463.
H123	关小红, 张立曼. (2006) 润肤止痒洗剂治疗特应性皮炎 57 例临床观察. 中国中西医结合皮肤性病学杂志 **5**(2): 113.
H124	宁晓红, 冻涛. (2004) 中西医结合治疗婴儿期特应性皮炎 84 例. 皮肤病与性病 **26**(4): 20–21.
H125	石庆荣, 曹晓平, 才吉甫. (2014) 他克莫司软膏联合中药汤剂治疗特应性皮炎的临床观察. 医药前沿 **(16)**: 325–326.

(*Continued*)

(*Continued*)

Study No.	Reference
H126	杨丽君, 韩玉涛, 张晓燕. (2010) 中药浴治疗对特应性皮炎患儿的疗效及对外周 CD4+CD25+ 调节性 T 细胞的作用. 四川医学 **31**(6): 783–784.
H127	杨雪源, 徐丽敏, 周爱民, *et al.* (2010) 含马齿苋及牛油果树提取物的医学护肤品辅助治疗特应性皮炎的临床观察. 临床皮肤科杂志 **39**(7): 460–461.
H128	张建民, 张勤, 高莹, *et al.* (2014) 肤乐霜治疗婴幼儿湿疹和特应性皮炎的临床观察. 中国实验方剂学杂志 **20**(12): 238–240.
H129	孙卫国, 张旭, 陈桂莲. (2011) 丹皮酚软膏联合地奈德乳膏治疗儿童特应性皮炎疗效观察. 中国中西医结合皮肤性病学杂志 **10**(5): 319.
H130	Bomstein Y, Rozenblat S. (2015) Treatment of atopic dermatitis with KAM-3008, a barrier-based, non-steroidal topical cream. *J Dermatolog Treat* **26**(5): 426–430.
H131	Park D, Tran NP, Duncan JM, *et al.* (2010) Complementary use of topical bitter melon for atopic dermatitis (AD): A case report. *Ann Allergy Asthma Immunol* **105**(5): A80.
H132	卜静波, 李冰玲. (2003) 四物汤加味配合外洗治疗异位性湿疹 42 例. 实用中医内科杂志 **17**(1): 49.
H133	才吉甫, 向红芬. (2013) 运用中药治疗儿童特应性皮炎在焉耆盆地的观察. 中国伤残医学 **21**(10): 257.
H134	迟慧彦, 郎 娜, 姚春海, *et al.* (2012) 龙牡汤治疗风湿蕴肤型特应性皮炎临床观察. 中国中医药信息杂志 **19**(5): 73–74.
H135	杜晓华. (2015) 中医辨证治疗特应性皮炎疗效观察. 医学信息 **28**(23): 74.
H136	付宏伟. (2000) 中药治疗婴儿期异位性皮炎 160 例. 中国中医药信息杂志 **7**(2): 66.
H137	胡学涛. (2014) 龙牡汤治疗特应性皮炎临床研究. 中医学报 **29**(11): 1674–1675.
H138	郎娜, 迟慧彦, 余远遥, *et al.* (2011) 龙牡汤治疗特应性皮炎的临床疗效评价. 中国中西医结合皮肤性病学杂志 **10**(6): 356–358.
H139	郎娜, 姚春海, 柏燕军, *et al.* (2007) 参归煎剂合湿毒膏治疗血虚风燥型特应性皮炎. 中国中西医结合皮肤性病学杂志 **6**(1): 22–23.
H140	李春莲, 郑秀利, 白彩萍. (2013) 中医辨证治疗婴幼儿特异性皮炎 82 例疗效观察. 山西中医学院学报 **14**(5): 54–55.
H141	李忻红, 田静. (2004) 补肾养血煎剂治疗儿童特应性皮炎疗效观察. 中国中医药信息杂志 **11**(11): 999.

(*Continued*)

(*Continued*)

Study No.	Reference
H142	李兴军. (2015) 中医药治疗特应性皮炎的效果. 中国卫生标准管理 (**19**): 139–140.
H143	刘汉长. (2006) 中医内外合治特应性皮炎疗效观察. 世界中西医结合杂志 **1**(3): 166–167.
H144	刘晓玲. (2014) 龙牡汤内服外用治疗特应性皮炎 38 例临床观察. 内蒙古中医药 **33**(15): 16.
H145	马一兵, 孙丽蕴, 王萍, *et al.* (2010) 健脾润肤汤联合外用甘草油治疗特应性皮炎脾虚血燥证临床观察. 北京中医药 **29**(9): 680–681.
H146	肖敏. (2008) 马齿苋汤合中药外用药治疗异位性皮炎临床疗效观察及血清总 IgE 水平测定研究. 成都: 成都中医药大学.
H147	赵一丁, 黄尧洲, 郎娜, *et al.* (2013) 田凤艳龙牡汤对特应性皮炎患儿 SCORAD 评分及外周血嗜酸粒细胞计数的影响. 中国麻风皮肤病杂志 **29**(1): 34–35.
H148	余鸿. (2013) 龙牡汤治疗特应性皮炎的临床疗效观察. 中国医药指南 **11**(26): 485–486.
H149	陈文展. (2003) 黛连油膏治疗异位性皮炎 26 例. 福建医药杂志 **25**(3): 224–225.
H150	李斌. (1994) 蜈蚣方治疗异位性皮炎 31 例. 吉林中医药 (**4**): 54.
H151	马一兵, 孙丽蕴, 王萍. (2009) 健脾润肤汤联合甘草油治疗特应性皮炎 36 例临床分析. 中国中西医结合皮肤性病学杂志 **8**(5): 310–311.
H152	王如伟, 刘洪浪, 李颂华, *et al.* (2011) 复方苦参颗粒对重度特应性皮炎 51 例的治疗效果. 中国中西医结合皮肤性病学杂志 **10**(4): 222–223.
H153	邢华. (2007) 朱仁康治疗异位性皮炎的经验. 中华中医药学刊 **25**(2): 229–230.
H154	姚高升. (1998) 中医药治疗异位性皮炎疗效观察. 北京中医药大学学报 **21**(6): 59.
H155	尤立平, 刘永生, 杨顶权, *et al.* (2003) 44 例特应性皮炎中医临床证候分析与辨证治疗. 中国中西医结合皮肤性病学杂志 **2**(2): 71–73.
H156	曾昭明, 潘伟军. (2007) 中药内服外用治疗异位性皮炎 47 例. 新中医 **39**(3): 56–57.
H157	(2009) 赵喆健脾消导汤治疗儿童特应性皮炎疗效观察及对脾胃功能的影响. 中国中医药信息杂志 **16**(7): 80–81.
H158	郑思维, 赵志国, 陈华, *et al.* (2011) 中药内服外用治疗异位性皮炎的临床观察. 中外健康文摘 **8**(5): 410–411.

(*Continued*)

(Continued)

Study No.	Reference
H159	周双印. (1989) 辨证治疗异位性湿疹 31 例报告. 中医杂志 (**12**): 36–38.
H160	Al-Khafaji M. (2009) Atopic eczema and the importance of resolving fire toxin. *J Chin Med* **90**: 36–46.
H161	Li S, Kuchta K, Tamaru N, *et al.* (2013) Efficacy of a novel herbal multicomponent traditional Chinese medicine therapy approach in patients with atopic dermatitis. *Forsch Komplementmed* **20**(3): 189–196.
H162	Zhou S. (1998) Clinical observations on the treatment of 182 cases of acute, subacute and chronic eczema with *Shizhen san*. *J Tradit Chin Med* **18**(2): 118–121.

6

Pharmacological Actions
of Frequently Used Herbs

OVERVIEW

Chinese herbs applied orally or topically may reduce the signs and symptoms of atopic dermatitis. The possible mechanisms of action of many of the frequently used herbs in randomised controlled trials have been examined in experimental studies. Studies have shown herbs to have anti-allergic and anti-inflammatory actions in animal models of atopic dermatitis and in *in vitro* studies.

Introduction

The actions of Chinese herbal medicine (CHM) formulas and individual herbs can vary according to chemical constituents and the combinations of compounds and herbs. As described in Chapter 5, CHM has demonstrated clinical effects for atopic dermatitis. Experimental studies can provide insight into the mechanisms of action of the herbs, herb extracts and constituent compounds used in CHM for atopic dermatitis.

The pathogeneses of atopic dermatitis are not fully understood. It is clear that atopic dermatitis arises from a combination of factors that include immune dysfunction, environmental factors, skin barrier defects and increased skin infections.[1] The pathological processes have been described in Chapter 1. Several animal models exist for atopic dermatitis, and have been described in detail by Jin *et al.* (2009).[2] The first model uses Nc/Nga mice that spontaneously develop atopic dermatitis on exposure to environmental aeroallergens.

The second model induces atopic dermatitis through repeated application of sensitisers to the shaved skin. Sensitisers may include allergens or house dust mites, haptens (small molecules that produce an immune response when combined with a larger carrier molecule) such as trinitrochlorobenzene (TNCB), dinitrochlorobenzene (DNCB), and oxazolone, superantigens such as *Staphylococcus aureus*, and food hypersensitivity. The third model of atopic dermatitis is in genetically engineered mice. In this model, mice are engineered to either overexpress cytokines such as interleukin (IL)-4, IL-31 and thymic stromal lymphoietin (TSLP), or lack selective molecules such as the aspartic proteinase cathepsin E. The sensitiser-induced model was used frequently in experimental studies described below.

Methods

This chapter provides a general overview of the experimental studies relating to the pharmacology of herbs and their constituent compounds for atopic dermatitis. The most frequently cited herbs used orally and topically in randomised controlled trials (RCTs) were reviewed by the research team, including expert dermatologists. Key herbs from the three categories were selected based on their clinical importance: Oral CHM (Chapter 5, Table 5.2), topical CHM (Table 5.13) and oral plus topical CHM (Table 5.23).

Key herbs used orally were *bai xian pi* 白鲜皮, *bai zhu* 白术, *dang gui* 当归, *fang feng* 防风, *fu ling* 茯苓, *gan cao* 甘草, *sheng di* 生地 and *yi yi ren* 薏苡仁. Key herbs used topically were *gan cao* 甘草 and *jin yin hua* 金银花. Key herbs from studies of oral plus topical CHM were *fu ling* 茯苓, *gan cao* 甘草, *bai xian pi* 白鲜皮, *sheng di* 生地, *yi yi ren* 薏苡仁, *dang gui* 当归, *bai zhu* 白术, *jin yin hua* 金银花, *long gu* 龙骨 and *mu li* 牡蛎. Some of the key herbs used orally in studies of oral plus topical CHM had also been identified from studies using oral CHM. The two key herbs that were unique to studies of oral plus topical CHM were *long gu* 龙骨 and *mu li* 牡蛎. *Gan cao* 甘草 was considered a key herb, whether used orally or topically. Experimental studies of *gan cao* 甘草 administered either orally or topically were reviewed for relevance.

The constituent compounds were identified by searching herbal monographs, high-quality reviews of CHM, herbal medicine encyclopedia,[3] materia medica,[4] and/or PubMed. PubMed and/or China National Knowledge Infrastructure (CNKI) were searched to identify experimental studies. The search strategy included the terms for each herb and their constituent compounds. Relevant data were extracted and a summary of the findings are reported here.

Experimental Studies on *bai xian pi* 白鲜皮

The root bark of *Dictamnus dasycarpus* Turcz. is *bai xian pi* 白鲜皮. More than 170 compounds have been identified from the *Dictamnus* species, with 92 of these found in *D. dasycarpus*.[5] Compounds include quinolone alkaloids, sesquiterpenes, limonoids, coumarins, flavonoids, triterpenes and steroids.[5] Of these, quinolone alkaloids and limonoids are the characteristic active constituents.[5] A wide range of effects have been reported with *Dictamnus* species, including anti-inflammatory, antimicrobial and immuno-suppressing actions.[5]

Research has examined the anti-inflammatory actions of *bai xian pi* and its extracts on contact dermatitis and in allergic disease models. Yang *et al.* (2017)[6] applied decoction of *D. dasycarpus* (DDD) in Balb/c mice with contact dermatitis induced by dinitrofluorobenzene (DNFB). Dermatitis symptoms of crust, scale, incrustation, pigmentation and petechiae were reduced with DDD, compared to controls. Erythema was also reduced with DDD, but not with dexamethasone as a positive control. Skin thickness was lower in mice treated with DDD and dexamethasone. Histological examination showed DDD inhibited epidermal hyperplasia, hyperkeratosis and spongiosis. Production of the cytokines tumour necrosis factor-alpha (TNF-α), IL-6 and interferon-gamma (IFN-γ) in the tissue lysate was lower with DDD-treated mice, compared to controls. Given the similar mechanisms, it is reasonable to expect that similar results would be seen for atopic dermatitis.

The methanol extract of *D. dasycarpus* has also shown anti-inflammatory activity.[7] Contact dermatitis was induced in Balb/c mice by repeated application of DNFB. Ear thickness and weight were increased after induction of contact dermatitis, both of which were significantly reduced with methanol extract. Dexamethasone was more effective than the methanol extract in reducing ear thickness and ear weight. Histology showed reductions in epidermal hyperplasia, oedema and spongiosis with methanol extract, compared to controls. Significant suppression of inflammatory cytokines IFN-γ and TNF-α in tissue was seen with the methanol extract. The study also examined mast cell degranulation, finding dose-dependent reductions in levels of histamine and β-hexosaminidase in rat basophilic leukaemia (RBL)-2H3 cells pre-treated with the methanol extract. In this study,[7] methanol extract of *D. dasycarpus* attenuated the allergic response by decreasing granulation of mast cells.

A second study by the same team examined this further.[8] Methanol extract of *D. dasycarpus* was found to act by regulating expression of intercellular adhesion molecule (ICAM)-1, also known as CD54. Intercellular adhesion molecule-1 is involved in recruiting cells to the site of inflammation. Again, the methanol extract was found to significantly reduce epidermal thickness and hyperplasia. Methanol extract also resulted in a slight reduction in TNF-α-induced ICAM-1 expression in inflamed tissues. In human keratinocyte (HaCaT) cells, methanol extract was not cytotoxic up to doses of 100 μg/ml. In addition, ICAM-1 surface expression in HaCaT cells activated by TNF-α was also reduced with methanol extract, and the levels of IL-6 and IL-8 were lowered. The anti-inflammatory actions occurred via preventing activation of the nuclear factor kappa-light-chain-enhancer of activated B cells (NF-κB) pathway by TNF-α. Furthermore, the ethanol extract of *D. dasycarpus* has also been shown to inhibit allergic responses.[9] Scratching behaviour induced by compound 48/80, histamine or serotonin in mice was reduced with *D. dasycarpus*. The reduction in scratching behavior was dose-dependent when itch was induced by histamine or serotonin; histamine release from rat peritoneal mast cells induced by compound 48/80 was also dose-dependently inhibited. The actions of *D. dasycarpus* may alleviate symptoms of atopic dermatitis.

Experimental Studies on *bai zhu* 白术

The dried root of *Atractylodes macrocephala* Koidz is the official species used for *bai zhu* 白术 in the Pharmacopoeia of the People's Republic of China (PPRC).[10] In the Japanese pharmacopeia, either *A. japonica* or *A. macrocephala* can be used.[11] The major bioactive components of *bai zhu* are atractylon, atractylenolide I, atractylenolide II, atractylenolide III and other sesquiterpenes.[12] Several of these compounds are common to *Atractylodes* species, albeit with differing concentrations.[13]

Atractylenolide I has been shown to have anti-allergy actions. The ethanol extract from *A. japonica* showed inhibition of 5-lipoxygenase (LOX) catalysed leukotriene in retinoblastoma-like protein (RBL)-1 cells.[14] Of the three major sesquiterpenes isolated from the ethanol extract, atractylenolide I had the strongest inhibition of 5-LOX. In the same study, Nc/Nga mice were pre-treated with the ethanol extract of *A. japonica* during induction of atopic dermatitis with TNCB. Scores for clinical severity and scratch behaviour were significantly lower with ethanol extract of *A. japonica* than controls, although no change in serum immunoglobulin (Ig)E was seen. Atractylenolide I was suggested to contribute to some of the anti-allergy actions seen.

Another compound of *bai zhu*, atractylenolide III, may also have anti-allergy effects via inhibiting TSLP-induced mast cell proliferation.[15] Human mast cell (HMC)-1 cells were stimulated with TSLP which increased IL-13 protein levels. Cells that were also pre-treated with different concentrations of atractylenolide III showed significantly lower levels of IL-13, and a dose-dependent reduction in IL-13 messenger ribonucleic acid (mRNA) expression was seen. Similar findings were seen for the inflammatory cytokines IL-6, IL-1β, IL-8 and TNF-α. Atractylenolide III could be an important anti-inflammatory agent for atopic dermatitis.

Anti-allergy activities of other compounds have been seen in related allergic diseases. Atractylone inhibited TSLP, IL-1β, IL-6 and IL-8 mRNA expression in HMC-1 cells stimulated with phorbol 12-myristate 13-acetate and calcium ionophore A23187 (PMACI).[16]

Cell viability was maintained with high concentrations of atractylone. The same study also examined the effect of atractylone on ovalbumin (OVA)-induced allergic rhinitis in mice. Atractylone reduced the rub scores and total IgE, compared with controls, and dose-dependently inhibited production of IL-1β and TSLP. The findings for atractylone may translate to other allergic disorders such as atopic dermatitis.

Experimental Studies on *dang gui* 当归

Dang gui 当归 is the root of *Angelica sinensis* (Oliv.) Diels. The key constituents have been summarised in a review by Wei *et al.* (2016)[17] and include polysaccharides, pthalides such as ligustilide (E and Z)[18] and organic acids such as ferulic acid, nicotinic acid and folinic acid. Z-ligustilide and ferulic acid are the markers for characterising the quality of *dang gui*.[19] More than 165 compounds have been identified in the plant,[19] 50 of these being identified from the root of *A. sinensis*.[17] *Dang gui* has been shown to have many actions, including immunoregulatory, anti-cancer, anti-inflammatory and antioxidant actions.[17]

Dang gui has been shown to reduce pruritus in DNCB-induced atopic dermatitis in mice.[20] Topical application of ethanol extract of *A. sinensis* significantly reduced scratching behaviour induced by DNCB, with a lower mean count of scratching bouts than mice treated with dexamethasone. Histological examination showed that the increased epidermal and dermal thickness induced by DNCB was attenuated by both dexamethasone and *A. sinensis*. Furthermore, *A. sinensis* significantly reduced dermal mast cell count and reduced serum IgE levels, compared with controls. Production of the cytokines IL-4, IL-6, TNF-α and IFN-γ increased after exposure to DNCB, and these were significantly reduced in mice treated with either *A. sinensis* or dexamethasone. This study showed both antipruritic and anti-inflammatory actions of *A. sinensis*.

Polysaccharides from *A. sinensis* have been shown to have immunoregulatory actions *in vitro*.[21] Polysaccharides increase proliferation in mice spleen lymphocytes. Production of T helper (Th) 1 cytokines IL-2 and IFN-γ significantly increased with polysaccharides, compared with controls, and the same was found for the Th2 cytokine IL-6 and for TNF-α. The effects were greatest for the 70% ethanol fraction of polysaccharides. The varying actions seen with the five fractions were attributed to their differing structural characteristics. Similar findings were seen in an earlier study,[22] with polysaccharides increasing total spleen cell, T cell and macrophage proliferation. Increased production of IL-2 and IFN-γ was also seen, and a reduction in IL-4 was found. This suggests that polysaccharides of *dang gui* regulate the balance of Th1 and Th2 cytokines.

Chinese medicine formulas traditionally include herbs in pairs to enhance the pharmacological actions. This was tested by Han and Guo (2012)[23] for the herb pair *dang gui* and *ku shen* 苦参 (*Sophora flavescens*). Herb extracts were evaluated for their anti-inflammatory and antibacterial actions alone, and in combination. Antibacterial activity was seen for the combination of *dang gui* and *ku shen* against five different bacteria, but *dang gui* extract alone did not exhibit any antibacterial activity. To examine their actions *in vivo*, endotoxin-induced uveitis (inflammation of the middle layer of the eye) was induced by lipopolysaccharide (LPS) injection. The combined extract inhibited production of IL-1β and TNF-α, while no difference was seen between *dang gui* extract and saline-treated controls. The model used in this study was not specific to atopic dermatitis, which may explain the lack of anti-inflammatory actions seen in this study compared to studies using atopic dermatitis models.

Experimental Studies on *fang feng* 防风

The roots of *Saposhnikovia divaricata* (Turcz.) Schischk. are the source for *fang feng* 防风. Forty-five compounds have been identified, or tentatively characterised, from *fang feng*, including chromones and coumarins.[24] A recent review of *fang feng* by Kreiner *et al.* (2017)[25] describes the bioactive compounds as coumarins, chromones, acid esters and acetylenes. *Fang feng* has various pharmacological actions, including immunoregulatory, anti-inflammatory and antioxidant actions.[25]

The potential role of *fang feng* in allergic disease was explored by Yu *et al.* (2015).[26] Allergic contact dermatitis was induced with DNCB in mice, and a series of experiments conducted. Ear thickness increased with induction of contact dermatitis, and was significantly inhibited in mice treated with *fang feng* extract. Serum IFN-γ increased with induction of allergic contact dermatitis *in vivo*, and was attenuated with *fang feng* extract. Conversely, IL-4 production in contact dermatitis mice increased. Similar findings were seen in lymphocytes from allergic contact dermatitis-induced mice. The study further showed that extract of *fang feng* inhibited naïve T cell activation into Th1 cells, and reduced the proportion of dendritic cells in murine lymphocytes. These findings suggest that *fang feng* extract modulates Th1 polarisation, and reduces activation of T cells and Th-cell differentiation.

A coumarin compound found in *fang feng*, praeruptorin A, has also shown to have anti-inflammatory activity in the croton oil-induced ear dermatitis model in mice.[27] The compound was applied topically after induction of dermatitis. The oedema induced by croton oil was significantly reduced by 22% with praeruptorin A, although other tested compounds including indomethacin produced a greater reduction in ear oedema.

Experimental Studies on *fu ling* 茯苓

Poria cocos (Schw.) Wolf is the official species for *fu ling* 茯苓. *Fu ling* is also known by many other botanical names including *Wolfiporia cocos* (F.A. Wolf), *Wolfiporia extensa* (Peck) Ginns, *Daedalea extensa* Peck, *Macrohyporia cocos* (Schwein.) I Johans. & Ryvarden, *Macrohyporia extensa* (Peck), *Sclerotium cocos* Schwein. and *Pachyma cocos* Fr.[28] *Poria cocos* (Schw.) Wolf is a fungus that grows on the dead and decaying wood matter of various *Pinus* species.[28] The bark of *P. cocos* is called *fu ling pi* 茯苓皮, the layer next to the bark is called *chi fu ling* 赤茯苓, the middle layer is known as *bai fu ling* 白茯苓 or *fu ling*, and the core with some wood attached (sclerotium) is called *fu shen* 茯神.[28]

A recent study of secondary metabolites of *fu ling* identified 147 compounds from the outer, inner and core parts of *P. cocos*.[29] Fifteen compounds were common to all parts of the 39 samples tested, suggesting that the chemical composition of each part is different. The two major compound groups are polysaccharides and triterpenoids,[28] and it has been suggested that triterpenoids are the most important compounds in *fu ling*.[30] Other compounds include amino acids, steroids, histidine, choline and potassium salts.[28] The anti-inflammatory, antioxidant and anti-cancer activities of *fu ling* are well recognised.[28,31,32] Other actions of *fu ling* include nematicidal activity, anti-hyperglycemic and antibacterial activity,[32] and immunomodulatory properties.[28]

Fu ling has been shown to have anti-inflammatory and immunomodulatory actions in atopic dermatitis. Bae *et al.* (2016)[33] treated mice with *P. cocos* bark (PCB) extract for 62 days using a murine model of atopic dermatitis. Atopic dermatitis was induced by applying house dust mite extract to the ear lobe. Mice treated with PCB had a lower ear and epidermis thickness than those who received a sham treatment, and a lower clinical score based on signs such as erythema/oedema, scaling/dryness and excoriation/haemorrhage. Histological examination showed reduced infiltration of Th cells, cytotoxic T cells, B cells, macrophages and dendritic cells, compared with sham-treated mice. *P. cocos* bark extract inhibited Th2-related immune responses in lymph nodes and increased the population of regulatory T cells (Tregs). The same study also conducted *ex vivo* experiments in CD4+CD62+L naïve T cells from mice. *P. cocos* bark extract significantly reduced IL-4, IL-17 and IFN-γ, compared with cells stimulated with T cell receptors. In addition, functional differentiation of Forkhead box P3 (Foxp3)+CD4+ Tregs was promoted with PCB. These findings suggest that extract of *fu ling* may suppress the immune system in atopic dermatitis.

A gene cloned from a purified protein from *P. cocos* (PCP) was found to induce a Th1 response in a murine model of atopic dermatitis.[34] When administered orally, PCP significantly reduced expression of IL-4 and IgE, and increased Th1-related cytokine production in splenocytes. Cell proliferation and expression of activation markers of CD4+ and CD8+ T cells were increased. The effect of PCP on Th2 signaling proteins was similar to controls, suggesting actions through upregulation of Th1 immune responses.

Anti-inflammatory actions of *fu ling* have been seen in other types of dermatitis.[35] In healthy human volunteers with irritant contact dermatitis induced by sodium lauryl sulphate, *P. cocos* was shown to decrease lesion score dose-dependently, compared with vehicle and untreated controls. Similar effects were seen for transepidermal water loss (TEWL). These effects were seen when *P. cocos* was applied in parallel to the induction of irritant contact dermatitis but were not evident when *P. cocos* was commenced once inflammation had already developed. From this study, the actions of *P. cocos* were preventive rather than therapeutic.

Experimental Studies on *gan cao* 甘草

Gan cao 甘草 (common name: Licorice) is sourced from roots and rhizomes of *Glycyrrhiza* species: *Glycyrrhiza uralensis* Fisch., *Glycyrrhiza inflata* Bat. and *Glycyrrhiza glabra* L.[36] Key compounds in *Glycyrrhiza* species are triperpene saponins, coumarins, flavonoids, calchones and other phenolics.[36] A recent review highlighted key pharmacological actions of *gan cao* including anti-inflammatory, antimicrobial, antiviral and antioxidant actions.[36]

Studies have examined the role of the constituents of *gan cao* in atopic, facial and contact dermatitis. Licochalcone A, a phenolic compound from *G. inflata*, was evaluated in an RCT for people with facial seborrheic, contact and atopic dermatitis.[37] Licochalone A was combined with 4-t-butylcychlohexanol, which acts as a sensitivity regulator, and compared with the synthetic corticosteroid triamcinolone acetatonide. Topical application of licochalone A and 4-t-butylcyclohexanol significantly improved the severity of dermatitis, TEWL, skin hydration and patient self-assessment on a 10-cm visual analogue scale. The intervention was found to be slower-acting than triamcinolone but showed greater overall improvements for erythema and skin hydration.

A key chalcone from *gan cao*, isoliquiritigen, was tested on atopic dermatitis-like lesions induced by DNCB.[38] Mice were divided into four groups: (1) vehicle; (2) DNCB alone; (3) isoliquiritigen alone; and (4) combination of DNCB plus isoliquiritigen. Lesions were induced in Balb/c mice by repetitive application of DNCB every three days from day six to 18. Lesion severity was scored for erythema/haemorrhage, oedema, excoriation/erosion and scarring/dryness, and scratch behaviour was monitored. Isoliquiritigen alone was similar to vehicle, suggested no irritating effects. Scratching behaviour and dermatitis score were significantly lower with isoliquiritigen plus DNCB, compared with DNCB alone. Serum IL-4, IL-13 and IgE levels were also lower with isoliquiritigen plus DNCB. Greater inhibition of the proinflammatory cytokines TNF-α and IL-6, and IL-4 mRNA in skin lesions was seen with isoliquiritigen. To test the effect of isoliquiritigen on activation of downstream immune cells, the Tamm-Horsfall protein (THP)-1 cell line was used. Lower levels of CD54 (a cell adhesion molecule), CD86 (a co-stimulatory molecule on antigen-presenting cells, APCs) and TNF-α were seen in cell lysate. Furthermore, isoliquiritigen abolished phosphorylation of p38 and extracellular signal-regulated kinases (ERK) 1/2 induced by DNCB, suggesting its actions are to suppress proinflammatory mitogen-activated protein kinase (MAPK) signaling pathways.

Glycyrrhizic acid (GA) has been found to have anti-allergy effects by regulating immune cells.[39] Allergy symptoms were induced using OVA in Balb/c mice. At high oral doses (100 mg/kg), the effects of GA on allergic symptom score and rectal temperature were similar to hydrocortisone. Expression of the Th2-related cytokine IL-4 by mouse spleen cells increased as the allergy was induced, but dose-dependently decreased with GA. At higher doses, GA significantly increased the Th1-related cytokine IFN-γ. Combined, this suggests that GA can modulate Th1/Th2 balance to reduce allergic responses.

Gan cao is used in many CHM formulas but is not without side effects and may interfere with the actions of some drugs. A review of the toxicology of *Glycyrrhiza glabra* found mild toxicity, and caution is advised when used during pregnancy.[40] The main side effects found from animal and human studies included in the review were hypertension and hypokalemic-induced secondary complications. Case reports have linked allergic contact dermatitis with use of a shaving cream containing *Glycyrrhiza inflata*.[41] Herb-drug interactions have also been reported with *gan cao* and its components.[36] These include, but are not limited to, interactions with cytochrome P450 enzymes, many of which are responsible for drug metabolism.[42] *Gan cao* constituents liquiritigen, isoliquiritigen, several flavonoids and arylcoumarins have been shown to inhibit p450 enzymes.[42] *Gan cao* should be considered with caution for people taking medication metabolised by p450 enzymes.

Experimental Studies on *jin yin hua* 金银花

Jin yin hua 金银花 is the flower from *Lonicera japonica* Thunb. More than 140 compounds have been identified from *L. japonica*, including essential oils, triterpenoid saponins, flavones, iridoids and organic acids.[43] Actions highlighted in the review of *L. japonica* by Shang *et al.* include anti-inflammatory, antibacterial, antioxidant, antiviral and anti-hyperlipidemic actions.[43] The anti-inflammatory actions have been examined in relation to atopic dermatitis, as well as actions related to the immune response.

The flower buds of *L. japonica* were found to inhibit histamine production.[44] In this study, high-performance liquid chromatography showed chlorogenic acid as the key component of *L. japonica*. An extract of *L. japonica* inhibited histamine induced by sodium laurate in human keratinocyte culture, compared to controls, with no effect on cell viability. No such effect was found with chlorogenic acid. Both were examined further to determine their action on L-histidine decarboxylase (HDC). L-histidine decarboxylase is an enzyme that catalyses histidine into histamine in a two-step process — initially HDC is translated to a 74 kilodalton (kDA) form, then further processed into the 53–55 kDa form which has stronger activity. Both *L. japonica* extract and chlorogenic acid inhibited 53 kDa HDC expression, compared with controls, while no effect was seen on the 74 kDa HDC. Thus, the actions of *L. japonica* may be either through inhibiting 53 kDa HDC expression, or through inhibiting HDC itself.

In an allergic contact dermatitis murine model, a water-soluble fraction of *L. japonica* was found to significantly reduce ear thickness.[45] Mice were treated before, and 15 hours after, challenge with picryl chloride to induce allergic contact dermatitis. The water-soluble fraction also reduced serum IgE and dose-dependently inhibited histamine expression, compared to controls. The pro-inflammatory cytokine TNF-α was also significantly inhibited, compared with controls, in a dose-dependent manner.

A key constituent of *jin yin hua*, chlorogenic acid, has also significantly inhibited expression of the proinflammatory cytokines IL-4, IL-5 and TNF-α in the lungs of mice with OVA-induced allergic asthma.[46] The same study also conducted *in vitro* experiments. In mouse splenocytes stimulated with LPS and IL-4, chlorogenic acid inhibited IgE production, compared with controls. Chlorogenic acid has also been shown to inhibit chemokine C-X-C motif ligand 8 (CXCL8) expression from eosinophil cultures, and in eosinophils-dermal fibroblasts co-culture.[47] The chemokine CXCL8 has been shown to be involved in atopic dermatitis. Luteolin is another compound from *jin yin hua* for which anti-allergy actions have been demonstrated. Inhibition of PMACI-induced inflammatory cytokines IL-8, IL-6 and TNF-α was seen in HMC-1 cells pre-treated with luteolin.[48] Inhibition was concentration dependent, with greater inhibition at higher doses. Luteolin may exert its effects through mast cell-mediated inflammation.

Experimental Studies on *long gu* 龙骨

Long gu 龙骨 is sourced from the fossilised bones of large mammals such as horses, cattle or deer (*Fossilia Ossis Mastodi*).[4] Resources of *long gu* are non-reproducible and are being depleted,[49] and research is being conducted to explore alternative sources.[50] Major chemical constituents include hydroxyapatite (a calcium phosphate), calcite ($CaCO_3$) and quartz.[4]

Few experimental studies were identified that examined the role of *long gu* in atopic dermatitis. Several studies have explored the effect of hydroxyapatite nanoparticles on the immune response. This may be due to calcium phosphate naturally occurring in the human body.[51] Rod-shaped hydroxyapatite nanoparticles were used as immunoadjuvants in a study by Wang *et al.* (2016).[51] The study also examined zinc- and magnesium-substituted hydroxyapatite due to the involvement of both elements in the human immune response. Cytotoxicity was negligible for all three nanoparticles in bone marrow dendritic cells (BMDCs). The levels of IL-4 and IFN-γ increased with all three nanoparticle types, and greater increases were seen with the zinc- and magnesium-substituted hydroxyapatite. In this study, both Th1 and Th2 immune responses were seen with a calcium phosphate constituent of *long gu*.

Hydroxyapatite nanoparticles have also been tested in normal and cancer cells.[52] Hydroxyapatite nanoparticles were found to decrease proliferation in human cancer cells, and to a lesser extent in normal human cells. Furthermore, hydroxyapatite was shown to increase the production of IL-1β, IL-8 and TNF-α in human peritoneal bone marrow dendrocytes.[53] While these studies have suggested hydroxyapatite may have actions related to immunity, there is a need to evaluate the actions of alternatives to *long gu*.

Experimental Studies on *mu li* 牡蛎

Oyster shell is the source for *mu li* 牡蛎. *Mu li* can be sourced from three species of the *Ostreidae* family: *Ostrea gigas* Thunberg, *Ostrea talienwhanensis* Cross and *Ostrea rivularis* Gould.[4] Major components include inorganic constituents such as carbonates, sulfates and phosphates, and organic constituents including pigments and proteins.[4] *The Encyclopedia of Traditional Chinese Medicine* describes three carotinoid compounds isolated from *mu li*, also known as *Crassostrea gigas*, including 3,4-Dihydroxy-3',6'-epoxy-1',2',5',6'7',8'-hexahydro-6'-methyl-16'-nor-β,φ-carotene-1',8'-dione, 3,6-Epoxy-5,3',4'-trihydroxy-12', 13',20'-trinor-β,β-caroten-19,11-olide and 3,4,3',8'-Tetrahydroxy-β,κ-caroten-6'-one.[3] However, a study by Maoka *et al.* (2005)[54] found these three compounds were from the edible part of the oyster. The literature search did not identify any experimental studies of these compounds.

Marine shells are generally composed of more than 90% calcium carbonate.[55] Calcium is naturally present in the human body, and plays a key role in triggering differentiation of keratinocytes.[56] Normally the transient receptor potential (TRP) channels of the canonical subfamily, in particular TRPC6, induce keratinocyte differentiation in response to extracellular calcium. In atopic dermatitis, TRPC6 is thought to be reduced, leading to impaired differentiation of keratinocytes. This may explain why *mu li* has been used for atopic dermatitis, although no studies were found that examined this pathway. Another source identified compounds cystatin A and gigasin from *C. gigas* nacre (the inner shell layer).[57] Search of electronic databases failed to locate any experimental studies relevant to atopic dermatitis. The mechanisms of action of *mu li* in relation to atopic dermatitis remain unclear.

Experimental Studies on *sheng di* 生地

Sheng di 生地 comes from the roots of *Rehmannia glutinosa* Libosch. Research has identified more than 140 compounds in *sheng di*.[58] Compound groups include triterpenes, monoterpenoids, phenolic acid glycosides, flavonoid glycosides, phenethyl alcohol glycosides, polysaccharides and lignans.[58] The constituents considered to exert its biological activity are iridoid glycosides such as glycoside A, catalpol and dihydrocatalpol, and *R. glutinosa* polysaccharides.[58,59] *R. glutinosa* has been researched extensively in experimental studies, with actions that affect inflammation, endocrinology and metabolism of glucose, as well as anti-tumour activity.[58,59]

Studies have evaluated the actions of *R. glutinosa* in house mite allergen-induced atopic dermatitis *in vivo*.[60,61] Sung *et al.* applied extract of *R. glutinosa* topically in Nc/Nga mice.[60] Atopic dermatitis was induced by repeated application of house dust mite allergen *Dermatophagoides farinae*. The severity of dermatitis was based on assessment of erythema/haemorrhage, scarring/dryness, oedema and excoriation/erosion. Treatment with *R. glutinosa* extract reduced dermatitis score at day 21 after induction of atopic dermatitis, compared with control mice. Ear thickness was also significantly lower in treated mice. Histological examination on day 34 showed decreased thickening of the dermis and epidermis, and less infiltration of inflammatory cells in treated mice compared with controls. Histamine release was lower in treated mice than controls, while total IgE was higher, suggesting that the actions of *R. glutinosa* extract in reducing clinical severity are independent to that of the effect of *D. farinae* on serum IgE levels. Furthermore, mRNA expression of the inflammatory cytokines IL-4 and TNF-α was lower in treated mice than in controls, and expression of Th2 chemokines (thymus and activation-regulated chemokine [TARC]; macrophage-derived chemokine (MCD); and regulated on activation, normal T cell expressed and secreted [RANTES]), ICAM-1 and vascular adhesion molecule (VCAM)-1 were lower in treated mice. Thus, the clinical actions of *R. glutinosa* extract occur through suppressing the actions of chemokines, cytokines and adhesion molecules.

A second study evaluated *R. glutinosa* using pharmacopuncture (injection of herbal substances at acupuncture points) for atopic dermatitis induced by *D. farinae* in Nc/Nga mice.[61] The actions of methanol and hydrodistillation extracts of *R. glutinosa*, and a herbal anti-inflammatory solution containing eight Chinese herbs, were evaluated. Clinical score was assessed based on the same parameters as Sung *et al.* (2011).[60] Clinical severity was lower in mice that received the anti-inflammatory solution, compared to controls, while hydrodistillation and methanol extracts were not different to controls. Mast cell count and serum IgE were lower in mice treated with the anti-inflammatory solution and the methanol extract. Levels of IgE were significantly higher in mice treated with the hydrodistillation extraction compared with controls. In all groups, expression of the inflammatory cytokine IL-4 was lower than controls.

Sung *et al.* (2011)[60] also examined the actions of *R. glutinosa* extract in keratinocytes (HaCaT cells) treated with IFN-γ and TNF-α. The extract of *R. glutinosa* was not cytotoxic and did not compromise cell viability. Dose-dependent inhibition of TARC was demonstrated with the extract, and MDC and RANTES levels were significantly reduced in treated cells. This suggests that extract of *R. glutinosa* alleviates atopic dermatitis by inhibiting infiltration of inflammatory cells.

The mechanisms of action of an ethanol extract of *R. glutinosa* have also been tested in RBL-2H3 cells.[62] Expression of the cytokines IL-1β, IL-6 and granulocyte-macrophage colony-stimulating factor (GM-CSF) was dose-dependently reduced in treated cells. Further, the effect of *R. glutinosa* on the high affinity receptor for IgE expressed by mast cells (FcεRI), was examined. Ethanol extract reduced mRNA expression levels of FcεRI, and prevented phosphorylation of Src and tyrosine kinase, thereby suppressing signaling pathways of mast cells activated by IgE/antigen. Therefore *R. glutinosa* appears to exert its clinical actions through suppressing mast cell activation through down-regulation of FcεRI-mediated pathways.

Experimental Studies on *yi yi ren* 薏苡仁

The seeds of *Coix lacryma-jobi* L. var. mayuen (Roman.) Stapf are the source for *yi yi ren* 薏苡仁. Also known as Job's tears and adlay/adlay bran, *yi yi ren* is an annual or perennial grass crop widely used as a food supplement throughout Asia.[63] *Yi yi ren* consists of four layers; the hull forms the outer layer, followed by testa, bran and endosperm/polished adlay as the innermost layer. Constituents of *yi yi ren* include lignan, benzoxazinoids, phenolic compounds (acids, alcohols, glycerides, ketones and aldehydes), flavonoids, polysaccharides, phytin, fatty acids, steroids and phospholipids.[64] Traditionally, *yi yi ren* has been used for skin conditions and inflammatory diseases.[63] Much of the recent research has focused on the anti-inflammatory and anti-tumour actions of *yi yi ren*, although other actions include antibacterial, antioxidant and hypolipidemic activity.[63]

Experimental studies have examined the role of *yi yi ren* in allergic diseases, with anti-allergy actions demonstrated. The effect of ethyl acetate fractions from ethanolic extracts of adlay testa on mast cell degranulation was measured as an indicator of immune dysfunction.[65] Mast cell degranulation in RBL-2H3 cells was seen in all four fractions of the ethanol extract, and was greatest with the ethyl acetate-soluble fraction. This fraction was taken through for further testing, and separated into eight subfractions. Four subfractions showed inhibition of β-hexosaminidase release (indicating mast cell degranulation), and also inhibited histamine release without cytotoxicity. Expression of the proinflammatory cytokine IL-4 was significantly inhibited at higher doses, with similar results seen for IL-6. Subfractions differed in their ability to inhibit inflammatory cytokines. Dose-dependent suppression of TNF-α was seen, and phosphorylation of ERK1/2 was suppressed. Finally, two of the seven phenolic compounds found in adlay testa (4-hydroxyacetophenone and p-coumaric acid) showed inhibition of β-hexosaminidase in RBL-2H3 cells. These findings suggest that at least two compounds of *yi yi ren* have anti-allergy actions which may be relevant to atopic dermatitis.

The same team conducted similar experiments using the bran and polished adlay of *yi yi ren*.[66] Again, no cytotoxicity was found and the ethyl acetate-soluble fraction provided the greatest reduction in mast cell degranulation by suppressing β-hexosaminidase release. Four of the nine subfractions significantly inhibited granulation of RBL-2H3 cells, and also demonstrated inhibition of histamine release. As was found for the adlay testa, subfractions varied in their ability to inhibit IL-4 and IL-6, with the greatest responses seen at higher doses; inhibition of TNF-α was also demonstrated. Four of the six phenolic acids separated from the ethyl acetate-soluble fraction were found to inhibit β-hexosaminidase release from RBL-2H3 cells.

The team then turned their attention to examine the actions of the ethyl-acetate fraction of adlay bran on humoral and innate immunity *in vivo*.[67] Using the OVA-immunised murine model, Balb/c mice were fed the ethyl-acetate fraction of adlay bran from weeks six to 12. Total serum IgE increased in mice immunised with OVA. This increase was suppressed in treated mice, both at high and low doses. Levels of IgE_1 and IgE_2 were also reduced in treated mice, which the authors suggest may indicate modulation of the Th1/2 balance. The ethyl-acetate fraction had no effect on phagocytosis, nor did it reduce natural killer cell activity, suggesting no influence on general immune function. The Th1 cytokine, IL-2, was increased in high-dose mice, compared with OVA-immunised mice, while the Th2 cytokine IL-4 was reduced. No effect was seen on another Th2 cytokine, IL-5. The anti-inflammatory actions of adlay bran ethanolic extract were found to suppress some Th2 immune responses.

The findings from the *in vivo* study by Chen *et al.* (2012)[67] were similar to those seen in an earlier study of dehulled adlay.[68] Using the same model as Chen *et al.* (2012),[67] Balb/c mice were fed an adlay-based diet for six weeks in three experiments. These included different preparations of adlay and different doses. Animals fed the adlay diet were healthy and their growth was not affected. Antigen-specific IgE was increased in OVA-immunised mice and was lower in adlay-diet mice. Levels of the antibody subclass IgE_{2a} were higher in adlay-fed mice than the control diet, while no effect was seen on IgE_1. Increased IL-2 production was seen, and IL-5 production reduced; no effect was seen on IL-4 levels. Adlay diet was seen to shift the balance from a Th2-dominant response to a Th1-dominant response.

Summary of Pharmacological Actions of the Common Herbs

For many of the herbs included in this chapter, experimental studies showed actions relevant to atopic dermatitis. Many of the studies showed anti-inflammatory actions in animal models of atopic dermatitis. *Bai xian pi, bai zhu, jin yin hua, sheng di* and *yi yi ren* showed anti-allergy actions, with the herbs reducing mast cell degranulation and suppressing histamine release. Anti-pruritic actions were shown with *dang gui.* This may be useful when considering formula selection or modification, as pruritus is a bothersome symptom of atopic dermatitis. Furthermore, immunomodulatory actions were seen with *dang gui, fang feng, fu ling, gan cao* and *long gu. Gan cao* and its constituents improved atopic dermatitis-like lesions when applied topically and showed anti-allergy effects when used systemically. An interesting finding for *fu ling* was that its anti-inflammatory actions were preventive rather than therapeutic. Of course it is not possible to predict who will develop atopic dermatitis in order to use this herb as a preventive treatment. However, this finding suggests *fu ling* is useful in the chronic stages between flare-ups. Further research is needed to examine this line of inquiry.

The biological actions of several herbs have been well researched, with many studies showing actions in atopic dermatitis and other allergic conditions. Two herbs have not received as much attention: *mu li* and *long gu*. *Long gu* is a non-reproducible resource which is being depleted, and research is ongoing to identify alternative sources that exert the same, or similar, clinical effects. Future research should investigate the mechanisms of this herb in relation to atopic dermatitis. It was more difficult to find information on the potential mechanisms of *mu li*. This may relate to the key constituent being calcium, which is a naturally occurring substance in the human body. Thus, the actions of *mu li* remain unclear.

References

1. Czarnowicki T, Krueger JG, Guttman-Yassky E. (2014) Skin barrier and immune dysregulation in atopic dermatitis: An evolving story with important clinical implications. *J Allergy Clin Immunol Pract* **2**(4): 371–379; quiz 80–81.
2. Jin H, He R, Oyoshi M, *et al.* (2009) Animal models of atopic dermatitis. *J Invest Dermatol* **129**(1): 31–40.
3. Zhou J, Xie G, Yan X. (2011) *Encyclopedia of Traditional Chinese Medicine: Molecular Structures, Pharmacological Activities, Natural Sources and Applications.* Springer, Berlin.
4. Bensky D, Clavey S, Stoger E. (2004) *Chinese Herbal Medicine Materia Medica*, 3rd ed. Eastland Press, Inc., Seattle, US.
5. Lv M, Xu P, Tian Y, *et al.* (2015) Medicinal uses, phytochemistry and pharmacology of the genus Dictamnus (Rutaceae). *J Ethnopharmacol* **171**: 247–263.
6. Yang B, Lee HB, Kim S, *et al.* (2017) Decoction of Dictamnus dasycarpus Turcz. root bark ameliorates skin lesions and inhibits inflammatory reactions in mice with contact dermatitis. *Pharmacogn Mag* **13**(51): 483–487.
7. Kim H, Kim M, Kim H, *et al.* (2013) Anti-inflammatory activities of Dictamnus dasycarpus Turcz., root bark on allergic contact dermatitis induced by dinitrofluorobenzene in mice. *J Ethnopharmacol* **149**(2): 471–477.

8. Han HY, Ryu MH, Lee G, *et al.* (2015) Effects of Dictamnus dasycarpus Turcz., root bark on ICAM-1 expression and chemokine productions *in vivo* and *in vitro* study. *J Ethnopharmacol* **159**: 245–252.

9. Jiang S, Nakano Y, Rahman MA, *et al.* (2008) Effects of a Dictamnus dasycarpus T. extract on allergic models in mice. *Biosci Biotechnol Biochem* **72**(3): 660–665.

10. Chinese Medicine Board of Australia. Nomenclature list of commonly used Chinese herbal medicines 2017. Available from: http://www.chinese-medicineboard.gov.au/Codes-Guidelines/Guidelines-for-safe-practice.aspx.

11. Shimato Y, Ota M, Asai K, *et al.* (2018) Comparison of byakujutsu (Atractylodes rhizome) and sojutsu (Atractylodes lancea rhizome) on anti-inflammatory and immunostimulative effects *in vitro*. *J Nat Med* **72**(1): 192–201.

12. Chen Q, He H, Li P, *et al.* (2013) Identification and quantification of atractylenolide I and atractylenolide III in Rhizoma Atractylodes Macrocephala by liquid chromatography-ion trap mass spectrometry. *Biomed Chromatogr* **27**(6): 699–707.

13. Cho HD, Kim U, Suh JH, *et al.* (2016) Classification of the medicinal plants of the genus Atractylodes using high-performance liquid chromatography with diode array and tandem mass spectrometry detection combined with multivariate statistical analysis. *J Sep Sci* **39**(7): 1286–1294.

14. Lim H, Lee JH, Kim J, *et al.* (2012) Effects of the rhizomes of Atractylodes japonica and atractylenolide I on allergic response and experimental atopic dermatitis. *Arch Pharm Res* **35**(11): 2007–2012.

15. Yoou MS, Nam SY, Jin MH, *et al.* (2017) Ameliorative effect of atractylenolide III in the mast cell proliferation induced by TSLP. *Food Chem Toxicol* **106**(Pt A): 78–85.

16. Kim HY, Nam SY, Hwang SY, *et al.* (2016) Atractylone, an active constituent of KMP6, attenuates allergic inflammation on allergic rhinitis *in vitro* and *in vivo* models. *Mol Immunol* **78**: 121–132.

17. Wei WL, Zeng R, Gu CM, *et al.* (2016) Angelica sinensis in China: A review of botanical profile, ethnopharmacology, phytochemistry and chemical analysis. *J Ethnopharmacol* **190**: 116–141.

18. Chen XP, Li W, Xiao XF, *et al.* (2013) Phytochemical and pharmacological studies on Radix Angelica sinensis. *Chin J Nat Med* **11**(6): 577–587.

19. Ma JP, Guo ZB, Jin L, *et al.* (2015) Phytochemical progress made in investigations of Angelica sinensis (Oliv.) Diels. *Chin J Nat Med* **13**(4): 241–249.

20. Lee J, Choi YY, Kim MH, *et al.* (2016) Topical application of Angelica sinensis improves pruritus and skin inflammation in mice with atopic dermatitis-like symptoms. *J Med Food* **19**(1): 98–105.

21. Wang J, Ge B, Li Z, *et al.* (2016) Structural analysis and immunoregulation activity comparison of five polysaccharides from Angelica sinensis. *Carbohydr Polym* **140**: 6–12.

22. Yang T, Jia M, Meng J, *et al.* (2006) Immunomodulatory activity of polysaccharide isolated from Angelica sinensis. *Int J Biol Macromol* **39**(4–5): 179–184.

23. Han C, Guo J. (2012) Antibacterial and anti-inflammatory activity of traditional Chinese herb pairs, Angelica sinensis and Sophora flavescens. *Inflammation* **35**(3): 913–919.

24. Chen L, Chen X, Su L, *et al.* (2018) Rapid characterisation and identification of compounds in Saposhnikoviae Radix by high-performance liquid chromatography coupled with electrospray ionisation quadrupole time-of-flight mass spectrometry. *Nat Prod Res* **32**(8): 898–901.

25. Kreiner J, Pang E, Lenon GB, *et al.* (2017) Saposhnikoviae divaricata: A phytochemical, pharmacological, and pharmacokinetic review. *Chin J Nat Med* **15**(4): 255–264.

26. Yu X, Niu Y, Zheng J, *et al.* (2015) Radix Saposhnikovia extract suppresses mouse allergic contact dermatitis by regulating dendritic-cell-activated Th1 cells. *Phytomedicine* **22**(13): 1150–1158.

27. Menghini L, Epifano F, Genovese S, *et al.* (2010) Antiinflammatory activity of coumarins from Ligusticum lucidum Mill. subsp. cuneifolium (Guss.) Tammaro (Apiaceae). *Phytother Res* **24**(11): 1697–1699.

28. Rios JL. (2011) Chemical constituents and pharmacological properties of Poria cocos. *Planta Med* **77**(7): 681–691.

29. Zhu L, Xu J, Zhang S, *et al.* (2018) Qualitatively and quantitatively comparing secondary metabolites in three medicinal parts derived from Poria cocos (Schw.) Wolf using UHPLC-QTOF-MS/MS-based chemical profiling. *J Pharm Biomed Anal* **150**: 278–286.

30. Wu LF, Wang KF, Mao X, *et al.* (2016) Screening and analysis of the potential bioactive components of Poria cocos (Schw.) Wolf by HPLC and HPLC-MS(n) with the aid of chemometrics. *Molecules* **21**(2) pii: E227.

31. Sun Y. (2014) Biological activities and potential health benefits of polysaccharides from Poria cocos and their derivatives. *Int J Biol Macromol* **68**: 131–134.

32. Wang YZ, Zhang J, Zhao YL, *et al.* (2013) Mycology, cultivation, traditional uses, phytochemistry and pharmacology of Wolfiporia cocos (Schwein.) Ryvarden et Gilb.: A review. *J Ethnopharmacology* **147**(2): 265–276.

33. Bae MJ, See HJ, Choi G, *et al.* (2016) Regulatory T cell induced by Poria cocos bark exert therapeutic effects in murine models of atopic dermatitis and food allergy. *Mediators Inflamm* **2016**: 3472608.

34. Lu YT, Kuan YC, Chang HH, *et al.* (2014) Molecular cloning of a Poria cocos protein that activates Th1 immune response and allays Th2 cytokine and IgE production in a murine atopic dermatitis model. *J Agric Food Chem* **62**(13): 2861–2871.

35. Fuchs SM, Heinemann C, Schliemann-Willers S, *et al.* (2006) Assessment of anti-inflammatory activity of Poria cocos in sodium lauryl sulphate-induced irritant contact dermatitis. *Skin Res Technol* **12**(4): 223–227.

36. Hosseinzadeh H, Nassiri-Asl M. (2015) Pharmacological effects of Glycyrrhiza spp. and its bioactive constituents: Update and review. *Phytother Res* **29**(12): 1868–1886.

37. Boonchai W, Varothai S, Winayanuwattikun W, *et al.* (2018) Randomized investigator-blinded comparative study of moisturizer containing 4-t-butyl-cyclohexanol and licochalcone A versus 0.02% triamcinolone acetonide cream in facial dermatitis. *J Cosmet Dermatol* **17**(6): 1130–1135.

38. Yu H, Li H, Li Y, *et al.* (2017) Effect of isoliquiritigenin for the treatment of atopic dermatitis-like skin lesions in mice. *Arch Dermatol Res* **309**(10): 805–813.

39. Han S, Sun L, He F, *et al.* (2017) Anti-allergic activity of glycyrrhizic acid on IgE-mediated allergic reaction by regulation of allergy-related immune cells. *Sci Rep* **7**(1): 7222.

40. Nazari S, Rameshrad M, Hosseinzadeh H. (2017) Toxicological effects of Glycyrrhiza glabra (licorice): A review. *Phytother Res* **31**(11): 1635–1650.

41. Wuyts L, Van Hoof T, Lambert J, *et al.* (2017) Allergic contact dermatitis caused by aftershave creams containing Glycyrrhiza inflata. *Contact Dermatitis* **77**(1): 49–51.

42. Qiao X, Ji S, Yu SW, *et al.* (2014) Identification of key licorice constituents which interact with cytochrome P450: Evaluation by LC/MS/MS cocktail assay and metabolic profiling. *AAPS J* **16**(1): 101–113.

43. Shang X, Pan H, Li M, *et al.* (2011) Lonicera japonica Thunb.: Ethnopharmacology, phytochemistry and pharmacology of an important traditional Chinese medicine. *J Ethnopharmacol* **138**(1): 1–21.

44. Inami Y, Matsui Y, Hoshino T, *et al.* (2014) Inhibitory activity of the flower buds of Lonicera japonica Thunb. against histamine production and L-histidine decarboxylase in human keratinocytes. *Molecules* **19**(6): 8212–8219.

45. Tian J, Che H, Ha D, *et al.* (2012) Characterization and anti-allergic effect of a polysaccharide from the flower buds of Lonicera japonica. *Carbohydr Polym* **90**(4): 1642–1647.

46. Kim HR, Lee DM, Lee SH, *et al.* (2010) Chlorogenic acid suppresses pulmonary eosinophilia, IgE production, and Th2-type cytokine production in an ovalbumin-induced allergic asthma: Activation of STAT-6 and JNK is inhibited by chlorogenic acid. *Int Immunopharmacol* **10**(10): 1242–1248.

47. Tsang MS, Jiao D, Chan BC, *et al.* (2016) Anti-inflammatory activities of Pentaherbs formula, berberine, gallic acid and chlorogenic acid in atopic dermatitis-like skin inflammation. *Molecules* **21**(4): 519.

48. Kang OH, Choi JG, Lee JH, *et al.* (2010) Luteolin isolated from the flowers of Lonicera japonica suppresses inflammatory mediator release by blocking NF-kappaB and MAPKs activation pathways in HMC-1 cells. *Molecules* **15**(1): 385–398.

49. Oguri K, Kawase M, Harada K, *et al.* (2016) Longgu (Fossilia Ossis Mastodi) alters the profiles of organic and inorganic components in Keishikaryukotsuboreito. *J Nat Med* **70**(3): 483–491.

50. Oguri K, Nishioka Y, Kobayashi Y, *et al.* (2017) Taxonomic examination of longgu (Fossilia Ossis Mastodi, 'dragon bone') and a related crude drug, longchi (Dens Draconis, 'dragon tooth'), from Japanese and Chinese crude drug markets. *J Nat Med* **71**(3): 463–471.

51. Wang X, Li X, Ito A, *et al.* (2016) Rod-shaped and substituted hydroxyapatite nanoparticles stimulating types 1 and 2 cytokine secretion. *Colloids Surf B Biointerfaces* **139**: 10–16.

52. Han Y, Li S, Cao X, *et al.* (2014) Different inhibitory effect and mechanism of hydroxyapatite nanoparticles on normal cells and cancer cells *in vitro* and *in vivo*. *Sci Rep* **4**: 7134.

53. Lange T, Schilling AF, Peters F, *et al.* (2009) Proinflammatory and osteoclastogenic effects of beta-tricalciumphosphate and hydroxyapatite particles on human mononuclear cells *in vitro*. *Biomaterials* **30**(29): 5312–5318.

54. Maoka T, Fujiwara Y, Hashimoto K, *et al.* (2005) Structure of new carotenoids with a 3,4-dihydroxy-beta-end group from the oyster Crassostrea gigas. *Chem Pharm Bull (Tokyo)* **53**(9): 1207–1209.

55. Hou Y, Shavandi A, Carne A, *et al.* (2016) Marine shells: Potential opportunities for extraction of functional and health-promoting materials. *Crit Rev Environ Sci Technol* **46**(11–12): 1047–1116.

56. Elsholz F, Harteneck C, Muller W, *et al.* (2014) Calcium: A central regulator of keratinocyte differentiation in health and disease. *Eur J Dermatol* **24**(6): 650–661.

57. Oliveira DV, Silva TS, Cordeiro OD, *et al.* (2012) Identification of proteins with potential osteogenic activity present in the water-soluble matrix proteins from Crassostrea gigas nacre using a proteomic approach. *Sci World J* **2012**: 765909.

58. Liu C, Ma R, Wang L, *et al.* (2017) Rehmanniae radix in osteoporosis: A review of traditional Chinese medicinal uses, phytochemistry, pharmacokinetics and pharmacology. *J Ethnopharmacol* **198**: 351–362.

59. Zhang RX, Li MX, Jia ZP. (2008) Rehmannia glutinosa: Review of botany, chemistry and pharmacology. *J Ethnopharmacol* **117**(2): 199–214.

60. Sung YY, Yoon T, Jang JY, *et al.* (2011) Topical application of Rehmannia glutinosa extract inhibits mite allergen-induced atopic dermatitis in NC/Nga mice. *J Ethnopharmacol* **134**(1): 37–44.

61. Kim MC, Lee CH, Yook TH. (2013) Effects of anti-inflammatory and Rehmanniae radix pharmacopuncture on atopic dermatitis in NC/Nga mice. *J Acupunct Meridian Stud* **6**(2): 98–109.

62. Kang KH, Lee KH, Yoon HM, *et al.* (2012) Rehmannia glutinosa pharmacopuncture solution regulates functional activation, FcepsilonRI expression, and signaling events in mast cells. *J Pharmacopunct* **15**(4): 32–41.

63. Kuo C, Chen H, Chuang W. (2011) Adlay (薏苡 yì yǐ; 'soft-shelled job's tears'; the seeds of Coix lachryma-jobi L. ma-yuen Stapf) is a potential cancer chemopreventive agent toward multistage carcinogenesis processes. *J Tradit Complement Med* **2**(4): 267–275.

64. Wu TT, Charles AL, Huang TC. (2007) Determination of the contents of the main biochemical compounds of adlay (Coxi lachrymal-jobi). *Food Chem* **104**(4): 1509–1515.

65. Chen HJ, Shih CK, Hsu HY, *et al.* (2010) Mast cell-dependent allergic responses are inhibited by ethanolic extract of adlay (Coix lachryma-jobi L. var. ma-yuen Stapf) testa. *J Agric Food Chem* **58**(4): 2596–2601.

66. Chen HJ, Lo YC, Chiang W. (2012) Inhibitory effects of adlay bran (Coix lachryma-jobi L. var. ma-yuen Stapf) on chemical mediator release and cytokine production in rat basophilic leukemia cells. *J Ethnopharmacol* **141**(1): 119–127.

67. Chen HJ, Hsu HY, Chiang W. (2012) Allergic immune-regulatory effects of adlay bran on an OVA-immunized mice allergic model. *Food Chem Toxicol* **50**(10): 3808–3813.

68. Hsu HY, Lin BF, Lin JY, *et al.* (2003) Suppression of allergic reactions by dehulled adlay in association with the balance of TH1/TH2 cell responses. *J Agric Food Chem* **51**(13): 3763–3769.

7

Clinical Evidence for Acupuncture and Other Chinese Medicine Therapies

OVERVIEW

This chapter describes the evidence of acupuncture and other Chinese medicine therapies used in three randomised controlled trials and three non-controlled studies. Overall, the evidence is limited and clinicians should use their clinical judgment regarding the use of these therapies.

Introduction

Acupuncture belongs to a family of techniques that corrects imbalances of energy and restores health to the body. Various techniques are used to stimulate acupuncture points, including:

- Acupuncture: Insertion of an acupuncture needle into acupuncture points.
- Acupressure: Application of pressure to acupuncture points.
- Moxibustion: Burning of a herb (usually *ai ye* 艾叶, *Artemesia vulgaris* L.) close to, or on, the skin to induce a warming sensation.
- Transcutaneous electrical nerve stimulation (TENS): Application of transdermal electrical current to acupuncture points via conducting pads.

Contemporary acupuncture clinical practice has retained several of the techniques described in classical Chinese medicine (CM) books. Acupuncture remains an important treatment option. Cupping therapy is another CM treatment that is commonly used in clinical practice. Cupping can be applied to acupuncture points or to specific body areas.

Previous Systematic Reviews

One review was identified in the English-language databases which evaluated the efficacy of acupuncture and related interventions for atopic dermatitis,[1] and a second review was identified from an Internet search.[2] No reviews were found in the Chinese literature. Tan *et al.* (2015)[1] proposed to review acupuncture, compared with placebo or sham interventions, using validated outcomes for atopic dermatitis signs and symptoms, and health-related quality of life, but no study met the inclusion criteria. The second review by Quan *et al.* (2015)[2] included five studies. The authors found that the effective rate with acupuncture/acupressure alone, or combined with other treatments, was better than the control groups, which included pharmacotherapy and Chinese herbal medicines (CHMs). The authors noted the low level of evidence when drawing their conclusions.

Identification of Clinical Studies

Search of English and Chinese databases identified 17,364 citations. The full text was retrieved for 539 studies to determine eligibility. In total, six studies met the inclusion criteria specified in Chapter 4. Three studies were randomised controlled trials (RCTs) and three were non-controlled studies (see Fig. 7.1). No controlled clinical trials were identified which were eligible for inclusion in this chapter. Interventions included acupuncture, acupressure, TENS and cupping. Characteristics of included studies and outcome data from RCTs are described.

Acupuncture

Three studies evaluated acupuncture (A1–A3). One was an RCT (A1) and two were non-controlled studies (A2, A3).

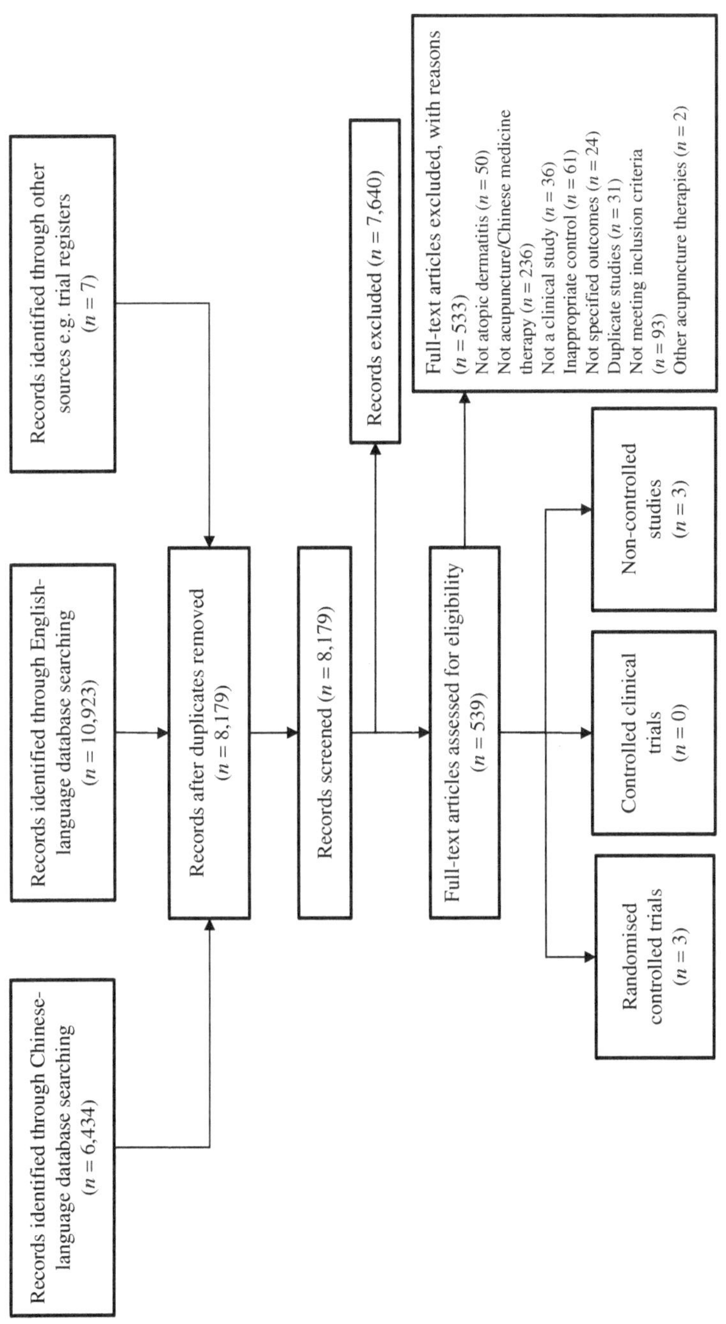

Fig. 7.1. Flowchart of study selection process: Acupuncture and related therapies.

Randomised Controlled Trials of Acupuncture

One RCT (A1) compared acupuncture with no treatment in ten participants. The study was conducted in an unspecified setting in Germany. Participants had history of atopic dermatitis for over ten years. Most participants were young, with a mean age of 25.2 years. The number of males and females was not reported. All participants completed the study. Chinese medicine syndrome differentiation was not described. Acupuncture was provided every three days for 33 days, with ten treatments administered in total. Acupuncture points used were LI11 *Quchi* 曲池, LI4 *Hegu* 合谷, ST36 *Zusanli* 足三里 and SP10 *Xuehai* 血海.

The quality of the study was moderate. The study used block randomisation to allocate participants to groups which posed 'low' risk of bias; however, insufficient information was provided about the method of concealing group allocation. The study was judged as unclear risk of allocation concealment. Neither participants nor personnel were blind to group allocation, posing high risk of bias for these domains. The outcome assessor was blind to group allocation, and the study was judged to be at low risk of bias for blinding of outcome assessment. No withdrawals were reported, and the study posed low risk of bias for incomplete outcome data. As neither a trial protocol or trial registration was identified, the study was judged to pose unclear risk of bias for selective outcome reporting.

The study evaluated three outcomes of interest to this review: (1) the SCORing Atopic Dermatitis index (SCORAD)[3]; (2) itch intensity using a visual analogue scale (VAS) and (3) adverse events. The effect of acupuncture on SCORAD and itch intensity was not statistically different to no treatment (mean difference [MD]: 15.80 points [–8.62, 40.22]; [MD]: –9.00% [–41.25, 23.25], respectively).

Assessment Using Grading of Recommendations, Assessment, Development and Evaluation

Using the Grading of Recommendations Assessment, Development and Evaluation (GRADE) approach described in Chapter 4, consensus was reached that acupuncture is an important intervention for which the strength and quality of the evidence should be evaluated. The expert panel identified that comparing CM treatments with topical corticosteroids (TCS), topical calcineurin inhibitors (TCIs) and emollients was clinically important. Outcomes selected for inclusion in summary of findings tables were SCORAD, itch severity, recurrence rate, health-related quality of life on the Dermatology Life Quality Index (DLQI)[4] and effective rate.

Based on the expert panel advice, six comparisons were identified. These included acupuncture compared with TCS, TCI or emollients, and acupuncture used as an integrative medicine with TCS, TCI or emollients compared with the same conventional medical treatments used alone. None of the included studies evaluated these comparisons. As such, we were unable to provide an assessment of the strength and quality of the evidence for acupuncture in atopic dermatitis.

Non-controlled Studies of Acupuncture

Two non-controlled studies (A2, A3) evaluated the use of acupuncture for atopic dermatitis. Both studies were case reports, with one study (A2) reporting one case report and the other study (A3) reporting two case reports. Chinese medicine syndromes were reported in both studies, which included Lung and Kidney defensive *qi* deficiency plus Blood deficiency leading to wind-heat (A2) and Spleen deficiency (A3). Four acupuncture points were described in both studies: KI3 *Taixi* 太溪, LI11 *Quchi* 曲池, LU7 *Lieque* 列缺 and ST36 *Zusanli* 足三里. One study (A3) reported a tapered approach to treatment, with acupuncture applied three times weekly for the first two weeks, twice weekly for the second two weeks, then weekly for the last two weeks.

Safety of Acupuncture

The RCT by Pfab *et al.* (2011)[5] reported that no adverse events occurred during the trial. Neither of the non-controlled studies (case reports) reported on adverse events.

Acupressure

One RCT (A4) compared acupressure with no treatment. The study was conducted in an outpatient department in the United States and included 15 participants with a median age of 34 years in the acupuncture group and 36 years in the 'no treatment' group. There were more males than females (10 males compared to 5 females). Chinese medicine syndromes were not described. Acupressure was administered by trained personnel and self-administered, with pressure applied to LI11 *Quchi* 曲池 three times daily for four weeks. Twelve participants completed the study, with one participant lost to follow-up in the acupressure group and two participants lost to follow-up in the 'no treatment' group.

The methodological quality of the study was moderate. The study used a computer-generated sequence to allocate participants to groups, and was judged as low risk of bias. The study was also judged as low risk of bias for allocation concealment, as consecutively numbered envelopes were used. Participants were not blind to group allocation, including the principal investigator who trained participants in the use of acupressure. The study was assessed as high risk of bias for these domains. Research staff who assessed outcomes were blind to group allocation, posing low risk of bias for blinding of outcome assessment. There was insufficient information provided about the reasons for participant withdrawal. Consequently, the study was judged as unclear risk of bias for incomplete outcome data. Similarly, a judgment of unclear risk was made for selective outcome reporting as no trial protocol was available.

The study reported on the Eczema Area and Severity Index (EASI),[6] change in itch intensity (VAS) and Investigator's Global Assessment (IGA), and adverse events. The authors reported that people who received acupressure obtained a statistically significant improvement in itch intensity and EASI lichenification score. No such effect was seen in people who received no treatment. The change in itch intensity, IGA and EASI lichenification score was greater in the acupressure group, compared to the control group. No adverse events occurred during the trial.

Transcutaneous Electrical Nerve Stimulation

One non-controlled study (A5) evaluated TENS in 46 people with pruritus due to atopic dermatitis, lichen simplex chronicus and chronic hepatic disease. As results were reported for each of the three conditions separately, the study was included for review. Ten participants who had atopic dermatitis were included, and received TENS to the itchiest and most distressing skin lesions. Chinese medicine syndrome differentiation was not described in the study. Treatment was applied every other day for four weeks, with a total of 12 treatments. The study reported two cases of mild erythema and one case of mild irritation and numbness with electrode placement.

Cupping

One RCT (A6) evaluated cupping therapy. The study was conducted in an outpatient department in China and included 50 participants. Participants were younger than in studies of acupuncture, with a mean age of 12 years. Twenty-seven participants were male and 23 were female. Participants had lived with atopic dermatitis for between 1.2 and 9.4 years. The study did not report CM syndromes. Participants in the intervention group received cupping to CV8 *Shenque* 神阙 daily for 30 days. Participants allocated to the control group received cetirizine tablets daily for the same duration.

The study was not free from bias. The report mentioned random allocation, but no further details were provided, leading to a judgment of unclear risk for sequence generation. Insufficient information was reported for allocation concealment and blinding of outcome assessors, and the study was assessed as unclear risk for these two domains. Participants and personnel were not blind to group allocation, which suggests high risk of bias for blinding. Data were available for all participants, and the study was judged as low risk for incomplete outcome data. No study protocol was identified, so the study was assessed as unclear risk of bias for selective outcome reporting.

In terms of clinical outcomes, the study reported on effective rate using the 2002 guideline.[7] Cupping therapy did not result in a greater improvement in skin lesions and symptoms than loratadine (risk ratio [RR]: 0.86 [0.66, 1.12]). The study did not report on adverse events.

Clinical Evidence for Commonly Used Acupuncture and Related Therapies

One intervention recommended in clinical textbooks and guidelines in Chapter 2 was evaluated by studies in this chapter on acupuncture. Acupuncture was evaluated in one RCT (A1) and two non-controlled studies (A2, A3). Two acupuncture points were used in all three studies: LI11 *Quchi* 曲池 and ST36 *Zusanli* 足三里. Both these points are recommended in the clinical textbooks and guidelines in Chapter 2. Furthermore, four more acupuncture points were common to two studies: LI4 *Hegu* 合谷, KI3 *Taixi* 太溪, LU7 *Lieque* 列缺 and SP10 *Xuehai* 血海. Evidence from the RCT did not show a statistically significant difference compared with receiving no treatment. In addition to acupuncture, clinical textbooks and guidelines included in Chapter 2 also recommend moxibustion, ear acupuncture, electroacupuncture, plum blossom needle therapy and *tuina* 推拿. No studies of these interventions were identified that met the inclusion criteria for this review.

Summary of Clinical Evidence for Acupuncture and Related Therapies

Acupuncture therapies appear to be used less frequently than CHM for atopic dermatitis. Two RCTs, which met the inclusion criteria, evaluated acupuncture and acupressure. In one RCT, acupuncture did not result in greater improvements in measures of disease and symptom severity, compared with no treatment, although the small sample size means it was less likely that differences would be detected. Acupressure was found to improve some measures of atopic dermatitis severity in one RCT, although no conclusions can be drawn from this about the efficacy of acupressure. The safety of these interventions in people with atopic dermatitis should be investigated in future research.

Both RCTs were small in terms of sample size, and methodological quality for both was moderate. Due to the nature of manual therapies, it can be challenging to blind participants and personnel who deliver the intervention. It is likely that this would have biased the results. Acupuncture interventions were delivered for between four to five weeks, which may not be a sufficient duration to see clinical changes in signs and symptoms. All studies reported using at least one acupuncture point recommended in clinical textbooks and guidelines included in Chapter 2, with LI11 *Quchi* 曲池being used in four of the five studies, and ST36 *Zusanli* 足三里 used in three. In this respect, it appears that acupuncture research is reflecting clinical practice to some extent. Practitioners may wish to consider these points for the management of atopic dermatitis.

Based on the findings presented in this chapter, there is insufficient evidence to support the use of these interventions in clinical practice. In planning future research, investigators should include the outcomes recommended by the Harmonising Outcome Measures for Eczema (HOME) consensus.[8] In particular, investigators should consider the use of the validated Patient-oriented Eczema Measure (POEM),[9] which is an important patient-assessed outcome. Further research with larger sample sizes will clarify the role these therapies may play in the management of atopic dermatitis.

References

1. Tan HY, Lenon GB, Zhang AL, *et al.* (2015) Efficacy of acupuncture in the management of atopic dermatitis: A systematic review. *Clin Exp Dermatol* **40**(7): 711–715; quiz 5–6.
2. Quan X, Chen D, Jiang Z, *et al.*, eds. (2015) Acupuncture for atopic dermatitis: A systematic review and meta-analysis. *7th International Conference on Information Technology in Medicine and Education, (2015)*, Huangshan, China. IEEE Computer Society.
3. Yu J, Kizhakkeveettil A. (2011) Acupuncture for the management of pediatric atopic dermatitis: Case reports. *Med Acupunct* **23**(1): 53–56.
4. Finlay A, Khan G. (1994) Dermatology Life Quality Index (DLQI): A simple practical measure for routine clinical use. *Clin Exp Dermatol* **19**(3): 210–216.

5. Pfab F, Athanasiadis GI, Huss-Marp J, *et al.* (2011) Effect of acupuncture on allergen-induced basophil activation in patients with atopic eczema: A pilot trial. *J Altern Complement Med* **17**(4): 309–314.

6. Tofte S, Graeber M, Cherill R, *et al.* (1998) Eczema Area and Severity Index (EASI): A new tool to evaluate atopic dermatitis. *J Eur Acad Dermatol Venereol* **11**: S197.

7. 郑筱萸. (2002) 中药新药临床研究指导原则(试行). 北京: 中国医药科技出版社.

8. Chalmers JR, Simpson E, Apfelbacher CJ, *et al.* (2016) Report from the fourth international consensus meeting to harmonize core outcome measures for atopic eczema/dermatitis clinical trials (HOME initiative). *Br J Dermatol* **175**(1): 69–79.

9. Charman CR, Venn AJ, Williams HC. (2004) The patient-oriented eczema measure: Development and initial validation of a new tool for measuring atopic eczema severity from the patients' perspective. *Arch Dermatol* **140**(12): 1513–1519.

References for Clinical Studies of Included Acupuncture Therapies

Study No.	References
A1	Pfab F, Athanasiadis GI, Huss-Marp J, *et al.* (2011) Effect of acupuncture on allergen-induced basophil activation in patients with atopic eczema: A pilot trial. *J Altern Complement Med* **17**(4): 309–314.
A2	Hobb J, Hopwood V. (2004) Acupuncture for the treatment of eczema: A case study. *J Chin Med* **76**: 48–53.
A3	Yu J, Kizhakkeveettil A. (2011) Acupuncture for the management of pediatric atopic dermatitis: Case reports. *Med Acupunct* **23**(1): 53–56.
A4	Lee KC, Keyes A, Hensley JR, *et al.* (2012) Effectiveness of acupressure on pruritus and lichenification associated with atopic dermatitis: A pilot trial. *Acupunct Med* **30**(1): 8–11.
A5	Ali B, Hegab D, El Saadany H. (2015) Use of transcutaneous electrical nerve stimulation for chronic pruritus. *Dermatol Ther* **28**(4): 210–215.
A6	龚磊. (2016) 拔火罐疗法治疗特应性皮炎 25 例临床观察. 基层医学论坛 **20**(08): 1094–1095.

8

Clinical Evidence for Combination Therapies

OVERVIEW

Using combinations of Chinese medicine treatments is common in clinical practice. Despite this, few clinical studies have evaluated the efficacy and safety of combing Chinese medicine interventions for atopic dermatitis. Evidence from one randomised controlled trial showed the combination of plum blossom needle therapy and cupping decreased atopic dermatitis severity on the SCORing Atopic Dermatitis index. The safety of combining therapies needs further evaluation.

Introduction

In clinical practice, it is common to combine different interventions to improve therapeutic outcomes. Combination Chinese medicine (CM) therapies are defined as two or more CM interventions from different categories administered together, for example herbal medicine plus acupuncture, or herbal medicine plus *qigong* 气功. Comprehensive searches of electronic databases and other resources identified seven clinical studies which met the inclusion criteria. These included one randomised controlled trial (RCT) (C1) and six non-controlled studies (C2–C7) (Fig. 8.1). Interventions included Chinese herbal medicine (CHM), acupuncture, plum blossom needle therapy, *tuina* 推拿 and cupping.

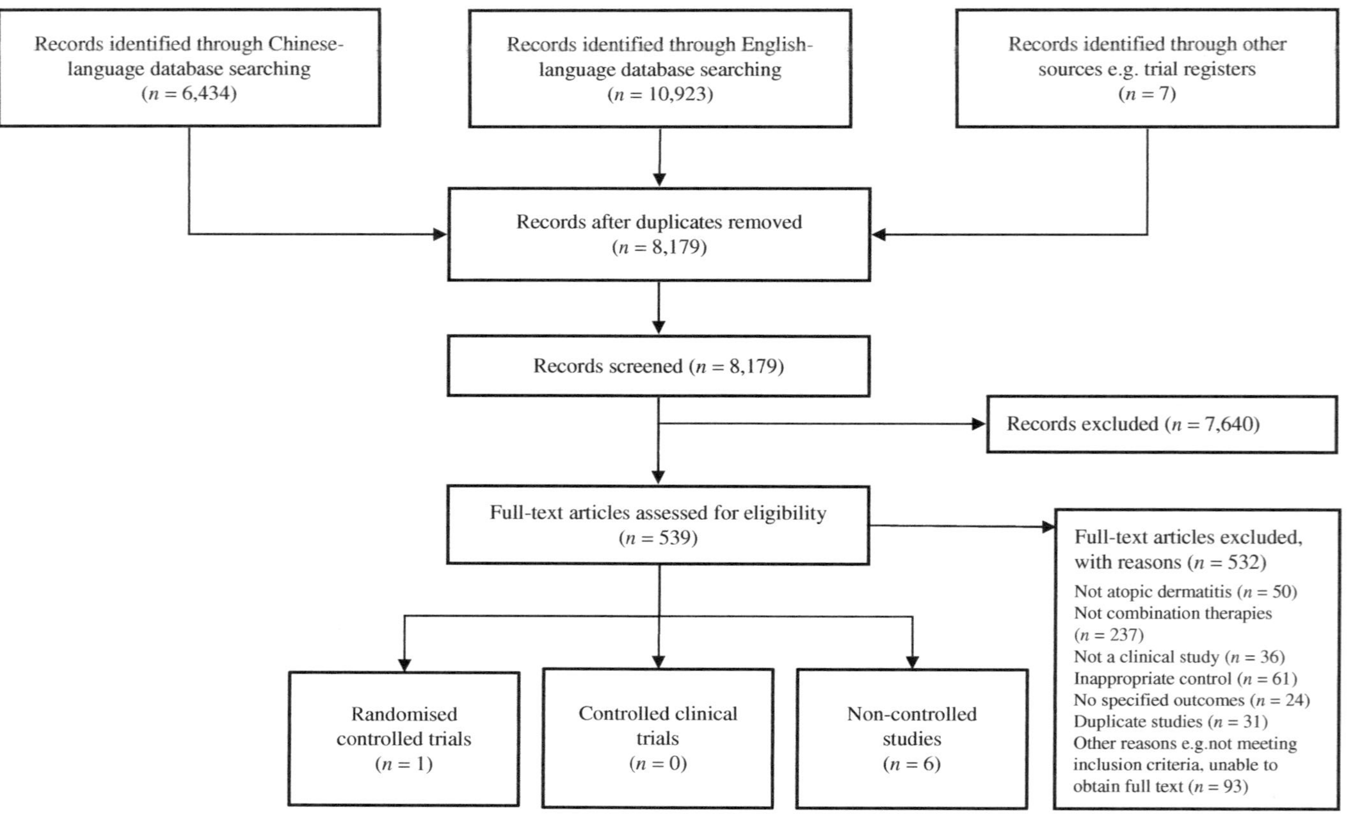

Fig. 8.1. Flowchart of study selection process: Combination therapies.

Randomised Controlled Trials of Combination Therapies

One RCT (C1), which evaluated a combination of CM therapies, was eligible for inclusion. The study was conducted in an outpatient department in China, and included 86 people with atopic dermatitis. The duration of atopic dermatitis ranged from three to 36 years. Participant age ranged from 13 to 39 years, and more females were included than males (48 females compared to 38 males). All participants completed the study.

The study did not report whether CM syndromes were evaluated. Participants in the intervention group received a combination of plum blossom needle therapy and cupping daily for three weeks. Acupuncture points were located on the back, and included GV14 *Dazhui* 大椎, BL13 *Feishu* 肺俞, BL15 *Xinshu* 心俞 and BL17 *Geshu* 膈俞. Participants in the control group received mizolastine slow-release tablets daily for the same duration.

Methodological quality of the study was assessed using the Cochrane risk of bias tool. A random number table was used to allocate participants to groups, posing a low risk of bias. There was insufficient information about how group allocation was concealed, and the study was judged as unclear risk for allocation concealment. Neither participants nor personnel were blind to group allocation (high risk of bias). A judgment of unclear risk was made for blinding of outcome assessor as no information was reported. As data were available for all participants, there was low risk of bias for the domain of incomplete outcome data. No protocol was able to be identified for the conduct of the study, which was judged as being at unclear risk for selective outcome reporting.

The study reported on the SCORing Atopic Dermatitis index (SCORAD)[1] and effective rate.[2] The SCORAD was lower among people who received plum blossom needle therapy plus cupping, compared with mizolastine alone (mean difference [MD]: −4.10 [−6.50, −1.70]). Analysis of effective rate did not show a statistical difference in the number of people who achieved a 30%, or greater, improvement in symptoms (risk ratio [RR]: 1.02 [0.95, 1.11]).

Non-Controlled Studies of Combination Therapies

Six non-controlled studies (C2–C7) were selected for inclusion. Two studies (C2, C3) described case reports, and four (C4–C7) reported on case series. Four studies (C2–C5) used a combination of CHM with acupuncture, one (C7) combined CHM with moxibustion and *tuina* 推拿 and one (C6) combined CHM with autohemotherapy. Of the six studies that evaluated CHM, two did not specify how the herbs were administered. In the remaining four studies, all used CHM orally and two combined oral with topical CHM.

Two of the six studies (C2, C7) described CM syndromes. One study (C2) reported the syndrome dampness with Spleen deficiency and Heart *shen* 神 dysfunction. The other study reported five syndromes: foetal heat and Spleen dampness, *yin* deficiency with Blood dryness, dampness-heat obstruction and stagnation, Blood deficiency with Blood stasis, wind-dampness and evil heat. Foetal heat is not a common syndrome in contemporary CM but is thought to relate to the mother having either a heat constitution during pregnancy, excess spicy and high-fat diet during pregnancy, or an unbalanced lifestyle or emotional factors during pregnancy. All studies used different CHM treatments, with no overlap in CHM formulas. Analysis of the herbs used showed *bai xian pi* 白鲜皮, *fang feng* 防风 and *sheng di huang* 生地黄 were most frequently used (five studies each). Other frequently used herbs are described in Table 8.1.

Three of the five studies that used an acupuncture-type intervention described the acupuncture points used. One study (C7) applied moxibustion to the affected area indirectly, through a moxibustion cake made with the herbs *bai xian pi* 白鲜皮, *fang feng* 防风, *she chuang zi* 蛇床子, *chan yi* 蝉衣 and *di fu zi* 地肤子. Acupuncture points ST36 *Zusanli* 足三里, LI4 *Hegu* 合谷 and LI11 *Quchi* 曲池 were used in two studies each. Other acupuncture points were used in one study only with no overlap.

Table 8.1. Frequently Reported Herbs in Non-controlled Studies of Combination Therapies

Most Common Herbs	Scientific Name	Frequency of Use
Bai xian pi 白鲜皮	*Dictamnus dasycarpus* Turcz.	5
Fang feng 防风	*Saposhnikovia divaricata* (Turcz.) Schischk.	5
Sheng di huang 生地黄	*Rehmannia glutinosa* Libosch.	5
Gan cao 甘草	*Glycyrrhiza* spp	4
Dang gui 当归	*Angelica sinensis* (Oliv.) Diels	3
Jin yin hua 金银花	*Lonicera japonica* Thunb.	3
Jing jie 荆芥	*Schizonepeta tenuifolia* Briq.	3
Ku shen 苦参	*Sophora flavescens* Ait.	3
Cang zhu 苍术	*Atractylodes* spp	2
Chan tui 蝉蜕	*Cryptotympana pustulata* Fabricius	2
Di fu zi 地肤子	*Kochia scoparia* (L.) Schrad.	2
Hua shi 滑石	Hydrated magnesium silicate	2
Huang qin 黄芩	*Scutellaria baicalensis* Georgi	2
Long dan cao 龙胆草	*Gentiana scabra* Bge.	2
Mu dan pi 牡丹皮	*Paeonia suffruticosa* Andr.	2
Mu tong 木通	*Akebia* spp	2
Niu bang zi 牛蒡子	*Arctium lappa* L.	2
Shi gao 石膏	Hydrated calcium sulphate	2
Tong cao 通草	*Tetrapanax papyrifer* (Hook.) K. Koch	2
Ye jiao teng 夜交藤	*Polygonum multiflorum* Thunb.	2
Zhi mu 知母	*Anemarrhena asphodeloides* Bge.	2

Note: The use of some herbs may be restricted in some countries. Readers are advised to comply with relevant regulations.

Clinical Evidence for Commonly Used Combination Therapies

Key clinical textbooks and guidelines described in Chapter 2 provide guidance on interventions that can be used for people with atopic dermatitis, but do not recommend which treatments should be combined. Several of the interventions recommended by key clinical textbooks in Chapter 2 were evaluated in studies included in this chapter. One RCT used the combination of plum blossom needle therapy with cupping; however, only plum blossom needle therapy is recommended in the textbooks described in Chapter 2, not the combination. This combination reduced atopic dermatitis severity on the SCORAD. Moxibustion, acupuncture and the formula *Xiao feng san* 消风散 have been evaluated in non-controlled studies.

Safety of Combination Therapies

Five non-controlled studies (C3–C7) reported on adverse events, with four (C3–C6) reporting no adverse events occurred. Three cases of dry skin at the site of moxibustion-cake application occurred in one study (C7) as a result of applying the intervention for too long.

Summary of Combination Therapies Evidence

Despite the practice of combining different interventions being common in clinical practice, relatively few studies which met the inclusion criteria evaluated the efficacy of this approach. Evidence from one RCT found that the combination of plum blossom needle therapy and cupping may improve eczema signs (SCORAD). Future clinical studies will provide more evidence on the efficacy and safety of various combinations of CM therapies. Interestingly, four of the six non-controlled studies evaluated the combination of CHM and acupuncture. This combination is commonly used in clinical practice; however, a comprehensive search of the literature did not identify any RCTs evaluating this combination. Accordingly, the potential benefits of CHM plus acupuncture in improving clinical outcomes remain uncertain.

References

1. (1993) Severity scoring of atopic dermatitis: the SCORAD index. Consensus report of the European Task Force on Atopic Dermatitis. *Dermatology*. **186**: 23–31.
2. 国家中医药管理局. 中医病证诊断疗效标准. 南京: 南京大学出版社, 1994.

References for Clinical Studies of Included Combination Therapies

Study No.	References
C1	傅祖伟,傅安. (2012) 刺络拔罐法治疗特应性皮炎临床观察 [J]. 新中医 **44**(2): 79–81.
C2	Chang JC, Gonzalez-Stuart A. (2009) Treatment of atopic dermatitis with acupuncture and Chinese herbal medicine. *Med Acupunct* **21**(1): 55–58.
C3	Kim MH, Yun YH, Kim KS, *et al.* (2013) Three cases of atopic dermatitis in pregnant women successfully treated with Korean medicine. *Complement Ther Med* **21**(5): 512–516.
C4	Salameh F, Perla D, Solomon M, *et al.* (2008) The effectiveness of combined Chinese herbal medicine and acupuncture in the treatment of atopic dermatitis. *J Altern Complement Med* **14**(8): 1043–1048.
C5	Wisniewski J, Nowak-Wegrzyn A, Steenburgh-Thanik E, *et al.* (2009) Efficacy and safety of traditional Chinese medicine for treatment of atopic dermatitis (AD). *J Allergy Clin Immunol* **(1)**: S37.
C6	候新珺. (2013) 荆防败毒散联合自血平衡免疫疗法在治疗特应性皮炎中的疗效观察. 中国保健营养 **23**(3): 1414.
C7	王敏东. (2013) 中医药治疗特应性皮炎 105 例临床观察 [J]. 实用中医内科杂志 **27**(11): 43–44.

9

Summary and Conclusions

OVERVIEW

Atopic dermatitis typically develops during childhood and may continue well into adult life. Conventional treatments are effective but preventing recurrence continues to be a challenge. Some patients seek treatment from complementary and alternative therapies, including Chinese medicine. This chapter provides a 'whole-evidence' analysis of the Chinese medicine treatments for atopic dermatitis. Evidence from classical and contemporary literature and clinical research is compared and contrasted. Implications for clinical practice and research are described.

Introduction

Atopic dermatitis is a common skin condition that can affect infants, children, adolescents and adults. Symptoms include skin rash and itch, and the course of the disease is characterised by periods of exacerbation and remission.[1] Basic therapy in the absence of lesions consists of patient education, basic skin care, and avoidance of irritants and allergens.[2] Topical treatments including corticosteroids and calcineurin inhibitors can assist for mild to moderate atopic dermatitis, while systemic immunomodulatory therapy and short-term systemic steroids are options for severe cases.[3,4] A key challenge in atopic dermatitis is recurrence, which contributes to patient burden.[5] Chinese medicine treatments may be of value in reducing disease severity and lengthening the time to recurrence.

This book uses a 'whole-evidence' approach to examine the Chinese medicine (CM) management of atopic dermatitis. Chapter 1 provides an overview of atopic dermatitis. Chapter 2 reviews key clinical guidelines and textbooks, highlighting key syndromes relevant to atopic dermatitis. Treatment options include oral and topical Chinese herbal medicine (CHM), acupuncture, electroacupuncture, moxibustion, ear acupuncture, plum blossom needle therapy and *tuina* 推拿. Examination of classical CM texts has identified topical CHM as an important treatment option, while few records of acupuncture-related or other therapies were found (Chapter 3). The methods used to identify, summarise and analyse clinical studies are described in Chapter 4. Analysis of clinical studies found oral CHM to be evaluated more frequently than topical CHM (Chapter 5). The evidence from CHM clinical studies shows some promising results for both oral and topical CHM, whether used alone or as an integrative medicine (IM) to guideline-recommended treatments. A selection of the most frequently used herbs in randomised controlled trials (RCTs) has shown various mechanisms of actions relevant to atopic dermatitis which may explain their positive effects in clinical studies (Chapter 6).

Compared with CHM, fewer clinical studies have evaluated acupuncture and other CM therapies (Chapter 7). Meta-analysis was not able to be conducted for RCTs, and currently there is insufficient evidence of the benefits versus harm of these therapies. More research is needed to examine the role of other CM therapies for atopic dermatitis. Combinations of CM therapies, for example using CHM in combination with acupuncture, are common routine practices. Despite this, few studies have evaluated the efficacy of these treatments used in combination (Chapter 8). Findings from one RCT have shown benefit for the combination of plum blossom needle therapy with cupping, but no clear conclusions can be drawn about the effectiveness of this treatment from a single study. The interventions combined in clinical studies in Chapter 8 were generally consistent with those in Chapters 5 and 7.

Chinese Medicine Syndrome Differentiation

Selection of treatments in CM relies on syndrome differentiation. Clinical textbooks and guidelines included in Chapter 2 describe five syndromes for atopic dermatitis, and an oral CHM formula to address each one. Syndromes focus on the concepts of Spleen deficiency, dampness, wind, heat, Blood deficiency and Heart fire. These concepts were also described in the classical literature included in Chapter 3. In particular, the concepts of maternal heat transferred *in utero*, wind invasion, Spleen deficiency, and Heart fire were found in citations considered most likely to be atopic dermatitis. The concepts linked with atopic dermatitis in classical literature are much the same as those described in contemporary texts, with little apparent variation in CM understanding.

More than one-third of included CHM clinical studies (66 studies, 40.7%) described syndrome differentiation, which was used as either an inclusion criterion or to guide treatment. Many of these reported multiple syndromes. While variation was seen in the names for syndromes, the key concepts were consistent throughout, and were aligned with those seen in Chapter 2. When syndromes were grouped according to key concepts, the most frequently reported syndromes across all CHM clinical studies were Blood deficiency and wind-dryness (18 studies), damp-heat (16 studies), Spleen deficiency with damp stagnation (eight studies), Spleen deficiency with Blood dryness (seven studies), Spleen deficiency (six studies) and wind-dampness encumbering the skin (five studies).

The most often described syndromes in CHM clinical studies were similar to those described in Chapter 2. Three syndromes named in Chapter 2 were found in CHM clinical studies: wind-dampness encumbering the skin, Spleen deficiency with dampness retention and Blood deficiency with wind-dryness. While no clinical study described the two other syndromes in Chapter 2 (heat accumulation in the Heart and Spleen and Spleen deficiency with Heart heat), several studies described the concept of Heart fire. Examples included hyperactivity of Heart fire and Liver fire, and relative predominance of Heart fire. Many of the concepts in syndrome names in clinical studies matched those described in Chapter 2, suggesting that many clinical studies were evaluating treatments relevant to key syndromes of atopic dermatitis.

Fewer clinical studies of acupuncture therapies were included, with two of the seven describing CM syndromes. These included

Spleen deficiency, Lung and Kidney deficiency *wei qi* 衛氣 deficiency plus Blood deficiency leading to Heat. The syndrome Lung and Kidney deficiency *wei qi* 衛氣 deficiency was described as a congenital deficiency. Neither the Lung or Kidney were included in syndromes in the contemporary literature in Chapter 2, although CM acknowledges the hereditary nature through prenatal *jing* 精. Other concepts seen in acupuncture clinical studies match those described in Chapters 2 and 3.

In studies evaluating various combinations of different CM therapies, two studies reported six syndromes. Dampness was described in four of the six syndromes, either alone or combined with wind or heat. Spleen deficiency was described in two syndromes, and concepts relating to Blood included dryness, deficiency and stasis. Blood stasis was not described in Chapter 2. However, Blood stasis can result from Blood deficiency, which was described in Chapter 2. So overall the syndromes stated in clinical studies of combination therapies reflect the key concepts described in Chapter 2.

While many studies reported syndrome differentiation, very few studies reported outcome results according to syndrome differentiation. One study that did so evaluated the same topical CHM formula for patients with three different CM syndromes (see 'Topical CHM' section in Chapter 5). For this study data were able to be analysed according to syndrome, but this was the exception to the norm. In other studies, data were usually reported in aggregate, meaning that it was not possible to establish efficacy according to syndrome.

Chinese Herbal Medicine

This section summarises the evidence from Chapters 2, 3 and 5. Chinese herbal medicine is an important intervention in CM management of atopic dermatitis. Treatments recommended in clinical textbooks and guidelines in Chapter 2 include traditional formulas and manufactured products for oral use, as well as topical creams and ointments. These treatments are targeted towards addressing underlying syndrome differentiation and/or to provide symptomatic relief. Chinese herbal medicine was the primary treatment option in citations from classical literature (Chapter 3), with 268 of the 271 treatment citations (98.9%) describing the use of CHM. There was diversity in CHM formulas, and topical application of herbs and formulas was more common than oral use (167 citations versus 97 citations, respectively).

The opposite was seen in the clinical studies included in Chapter 5, where more studies evaluated oral CHM (51 studies) compared to topical CHM (38 studies) and the combination of oral plus topical CHM (33 studies). Many of the formulas were investigator-developed, possibly modifications of traditional formulas, although this is very difficult to determine. This was also found in the classical literature, with many unnamed formulas that were described in terms of herb ingredients.

The number of RCTs that evaluated CHM alone and as an IM to guideline-recommended treatments was similar for oral CHM (25 and 27 studies, respectively) and topical CHM (14 and 11 studies, respectively). When the combination of oral and topical CHM was evaluated, 17 of the 18 studies used CHM alone. The reasons for this are unclear but may relate to the greater onus on the participants to adhere to oral and topical CHM, as well as conventional medication, or the necessity of a more complicated clinical trial design.

Meta-analyses showed benefits for several outcomes. When used alone, oral CHM produced a greater reduction in SCORing Atopic Dermatitis index (SCORAD),[6] indicating better clinical outcomes, than pharmacotherapy (Chapter 5, Table 5.4). Oral CHM also reduced the chance of relapse within six months, and improved the effective rate compared to pharmacotherapy. As an IM to pharmacotherapy, oral CHM improved clinical signs on SCORAD, reduced severity of itch and sleep disruption on the visual analogue scale (VAS), reduced recurrence within six months and improved effective rate (Chapter 5, Table 5.8). Further benefits were seen when oral CHM was combined with narrow band ultraviolet B (NB-UVB) phototherapy in terms of clinical signs.

No benefits were seen in meta-analyses when topical CHM was used alone. When combined with pharmacotherapy, topical CHM improved atopic dermatitis severity on SCORAD and reduced the chance of recurrence within six months (Chapter 5, Table 5.16). Using oral and topical CHM together improved results on SCORAD and reduced itch severity (Chapter 5, Table 5.26). Furthermore, oral plus topical CHM reduced the chance of recurrence in the longer term (six months or more). These findings show promising evidence for CHM; however, the results need to be interpreted in light of the quality of the evidence.

Consultation with experts in dermatology and CM identified several important clinical questions. Assessment of the strength and quality of evidence was conducted using the Grading of Recommendations Assessment, Development and Evaluation (GRADE). For many clinically important comparisons there were either no studies that evaluated the comparison, or no studies that reported on the outcomes judged to be clinically important. As such, GRADE assessments were able to be conducted for five comparisons: (1) oral CHM as an IM versus topical corticosteroids (TCS); (2) topical CHM versus TCS; (3) topical CHM as an integrative medicine (IM) versus TCS; (4) topical CHM as an IM versus topical calcineurin inhibitors (TCI) and (5) oral plus topical CHM versus TCS.

The evidence for oral CHM as an IM, compared to TCS, comes from low-quality evidence, and found no statistically significant difference between groups in effective rate (30% improvement in symptoms). Moderate-quality evidence showed no benefit of topical CHM alone, compared with TCS (Chapter 5, Table 5.18). For the same comparison, there was low-quality evidence that topical CHM improved itch severity, but topical CHM was not statistically different to TCS in terms of the effective rate (30% improvement in symptoms).

Evidence showed topical CHM as an IM produced greater improvements in SCORAD and reduced the chance of recurrence compared to TCS alone, but the quality of evidence was low (Chapter 5, Table 5.19). As a result, we are less certain that these studies show a true treatment effect. Compared with TCI alone, topical CHM plus

TCI reduced quality of life scores on the Dermatology Life Quality Index (DLQI), indicating an improvement in health-related quality of life (Chapter 5, Table 5.20). Topical CHM as an IM was no different to TCI alone in reducing recurrence or improving the effective rate, and the quality of evidence for these outcomes was judged as low.

CHM is not without side effects. In studies where oral CHM was administered, adverse events were generally mild and tended to be gastrointestinal in nature. Adverse events with topical CHM were less common than with guideline-recommended pharmacotherapy, and included a mix of gastrointestinal and dermatological events.

Chinese Herbal Medicine Formulas in Key Clinical Guidelines and Textbooks, Classical Literature and Clinical Studies

Chinese herbal medicine formulas are recommended in clinical guidelines and textbooks in Chapter 2, and are a prominent feature in the management of atopic dermatitis in classical CM texts. Furthermore, many clinical studies have evaluated traditional formulas, investigator-developed formulas and unnamed formulas. This section summarises the formulas used across these different types of evidence.

Assessing whether formulas were used across different evidence types is limited to searching for the name of the formula, regardless of ingredients used. Unnamed formulas were excluded from this analysis. It is possible that formulas with the same, or similar, herb ingredients, but with different formula names were included but were not counted in frequency analysis. In addition, the use of investigator-developed formulas in clinical studies was common, and some of these may have included the same ingredients as traditional formulas. Such instances would not have been identified as a use of a traditional formula. As assessment of similarity of formulas is complex and was not undertaken, the actual number for each listed formula may be higher than reported below.

Table 9.1 summarises the frequency of oral CHM formulas that have been recommended in clinical texts and guidelines included in

Table 9.1. Summary of Oral Chinese Herbal Medicine Traditional Formulas

Formula Name	Clinical Guidelines and Textbooks (Chapter 2)	Classical Literature (Chapter 3) (No. of Citations)	Clinical Studies in Chapter 5[a] (No. of Studies)			Combination Therapies (Chapter 8) (No. of Studies)
			RCTs	CCTs	Non-controlled Studies	
Chu shi wei ling tang 除湿胃苓汤	No	0	2	0	0	0
Modified Dang gui yin zi 当归饮子加减	Yes	9	4	0	3	0
Long dan xie gan tang 龙胆泻肝汤	No	0	2	0	1	0
Pei tu qing xin fang 培土清心方	Yes	0	1	0	4	0
San xin dao chi yin/san 三心导赤饮/散	Yes	0	0	0	1	0
Si wu tang 四物汤	No	3	2	0	1	0
Modified *Xiao er hua shi tang* 小儿化湿汤加减	Yes	0	0	0	1	0
Modified *Xiao feng san* 消风散加减	Yes	13	4	0	4	2

[a]Includes studies where oral CHM was combined with topical CHM.
Abbreviations: RCTs, randomised controlled trials; CCTs, controlled clinical trials.

Chapter 2, and formulas that have been evaluated in two or more RCTs. Formulas were included irrespective of whether modifications were made. Five traditional CHM formulas for oral use were included in Chapter 2, all of which have been evaluated or used in at least one clinical study (Table 9.1).

Two oral CHM traditional formulas have consistent use across the different types of evidence. Both *Dang gui yin zi* 当归饮子加减 and *Xiao feng san* 消风散加减 have been recommended in clinical guidelines in Chapter 2, were found in classical literature and have been evaluated in clinical studies. Their long history of use suggests that these formulas can be beneficial for people with atopic dermatitis. Whilst both were used in four RCTs, they were often combined with other oral CHM formulas, used as an IM, or did not report outcomes in a way that permitted re-analysis. Regardless, meta-analysis of the results was not able to be conducted for these formulas, and the potential benefits described in Chapter 5 are based on single studies only.

Clinical studies have evaluated formulas other than those recommended in clinical guidelines. Three formulas tested in two or more RCTs were included in Chapter 2: *Chu shi wei ling tang* 除湿胃苓汤, *Long dan xie gan tang* 龙胆泻肝汤 and *Si wu tang* 四物汤. *Si wu tang* 四物汤 was also identified in classical literature citations related to atopic dermatitis. This formula is used to tonify Blood, which aligns with the aetiology and pathogenesis described in the contemporary literature in Chapter 2 and classical literature in Chapter 3.

Clinical guidelines also recommend manufactured products for the various syndrome differentiations (Table 9.2). Some commercially available products were manufactured forms of traditional formulas. For example, *Fang feng tong sheng wan* 防风通圣丸 is recommended by guidelines in Chapter 2 to treat the syndrome wind-dampness encumbering the skin. This formulation was described in the three citations from the Qing dynasty, with these three citations judged 'most likely' to be atopic dermatitis. *Fang feng tong sheng wan* 防风通圣丸 was the only manufactured product from Chapter 2 that was found in the classical literature, but interestingly was not evaluated in clinical studies included in Chapters 5 and 8.

Some products are extracts of herbs, such as *Fu fang gan cao suan gan pian* (compound glycyrrhizin) 复方甘草酸苷片 from *gan cao* 甘草. These were not likely to be found in classical literature. Clinical evidence was sparse for other oral CHM manufactured products described in Chapter 2, with two products not being found in classical literature nor evaluated in clinical studies: *Shi du qing* capsule 湿毒清胶囊 and *Xiao er qi xing cha ke li* (granules) 小儿七星茶颗粒.

Topical CHM treatments can complement the use of oral formulas. Of the eight topical CHM formulas described in Chapter 2, clinical evidence was available for only one: *Huang lian* ointment 黄连软膏 (Table 9.3). *Huang lian* ointment 黄连软膏 was found in all

Table 9.2. Summary of Oral Chinese Herbal Medicine Manufactured Products

Product Name	Clinical Guidelines and Textbooks (Chapter 2)	Classical Literature (Chapter 3) (No. of Citations)	Clinical Studies in Chapter 5[a] (No. of Studies)			Combination Therapies (Chapter 8) (No. of Studies)
			RCTs	**CCTs**	**Non-controlled Studies**	
Fang feng tong sheng wan 防风通圣丸	Yes	3[b]	0	0	0	0
Qi pi wan/Qi pi wan ke li ji 启脾丸/启脾丸颗粒	Yes	0	1	0	0	0
Run zao zhi yang capsule 润燥止痒胶囊	Yes	0	0	0	1	0
Shen ling bai zhu san (wan) 参苓白术散 (丸)	Yes	0	1	0	0	0
Shi du qing capsule 湿毒清胶囊	Yes	0	0	0	0	0
Xiao er qi xing cha ke li 小儿七星茶颗粒	Yes	0	0	0	0	0
Fu fang gan cao suan gan pian 复方甘草酸苷片	No	0	4	1	1	0

[a]Includes studies where oral CHM was combined with topical CHM.
[b]Fang feng tong sheng san 防风通圣散.
Abbreviations: RCTs, randomised controlled trials; CCTs, controlled clinical trials.

different types of evidence i.e., recommended in guidelines in Chapter 2, described in five citations in classical literature in Chapter 3 and evaluated in two clinical studies in Chapter 5. One of the key actions of *huang lian* 黄连 is to clear heat when applied topically,[7] making this herb an important choice for atopic dermatitis. For the remaining seven topical CHM treatments, there was no evidence of use from citations included in classical literature, nor were any clinical studies included in Chapters 5 and 9. The evidence to support the use of these treatments in clinical practice is lacking. Practitioners should consider the potential risk and benefits for these

Table 9.3. Summary of Topical Chinese Herbal Medicine Formulas

Formula Name	Clinical Guidelines and Textbooks (Chapter 2)	Classical Literature (Chapter 3) (No. of Citations)	Clinical Studies in Chapter 5[a] (No. of Studies)			Combination Therapies (Chapter 8) (No. of Studies)
			RCTs	CCTs	Non-controlled Studies	
Chuan bai zhi yang lotion 川百止痒洗剂	Yes	0	0	0	0	0
Fu fang huang bai lotion 复方黄柏液	Yes	0	0	0	0	0
Fu fang she zhi ointment 复方蛇脂软膏	Yes	0	0	0	0	0
Hei dou liu you ointment 黑豆馏油软膏	Yes	0	0	0	0	0
Huang bai cream 黄柏霜	Yes	0	0	0	0	0
Huang lian ointment 黄连软膏	Yes	5	1	0	1	0
Jin huang gao 金黄膏	No	0	2	0	0	0
Pi fu kang lotion 皮肤康洗液	Yes	0	0	0	0	0
Qing peng cream 青鹏乳膏	Yes	0	0	0	0	0

[a]Includes studies where oral CHM was combined with topical CHM.

Abbreviations: RCTs, randomised controlled trials; CCTs, controlled clinical trials.

CHM treatments according to the CM syndrome and clinical presentation of each individual patient.

One topical CHM was not recommended in clinical guidelines but was evaluated in two RCTs: *Jin huang gao* 金黄膏. Meta-analysis was not able to be conducted due to differences in comparators and outcomes reported. While on the surface this may suggest that *Jin huang gao* 金黄膏 is an important formula that has received research attention, closer examination showed both RCTs were conducted by the same research team. So this formulation may have no more or less importance than any other topical CHM treatment.

Named traditional CHM formulas recommended for oral use in clinical guidelines and textbooks were evaluated in more clinical trials than manufactured products. It should be noted that many clinical studies used modified versions of traditional formulas, and any evidence of efficacy for modified formulas may not translate to evidence for the traditional formula. Many investigators developed their own formulas, which may have been based on traditional formulas. This may explain why the number of studies evaluating traditional formulas included in Chapter 2 was low. Comparatively fewer studies evaluated manufactured products that were included in Chapter 2. This may reflect practitioner's preferences to modify formulas to optimise treatment response or may be due to pre-existing evidence for commercially available products.

Of note, few clinical studies evaluated the topical treatments included in Chapter 2. While the number of citations describing topical CHM in classical literature outweighed oral CHM use, the opposite was true for clinical studies. The fact that few clinical guideline-recommended topical CHM treatments have been evaluated in clinical studies may reflect greater diversity, and therefore lower frequency, of topical treatments.

Acupuncture and Other Chinese Medicine Therapies

This section summarises the evidence from Chapters 2, 3 and 7. Acupuncture and similar therapies provide an additional treatment option for CM practitioners treating atopic dermatitis. Five acupuncture therapies are recommended in the key clinical textbooks and clinical practice guidelines included in Chapter 2: (1) acupuncture; (2) moxibustion; (3) ear acupuncture; (4) electroacupuncture; and (5) plum blossom needle therapy. One citation from the Qing dynasty described the use of acupuncture in classical literature (see Chapter 3). This suggests that acupuncture was not the first-choice treatment for atopic dermatitis. Indeed, similar findings have been found for other skin conditions in books in this series.[8,9]

Acupuncture was the sole 'acupuncture therapy' intervention recommended in clinical guidelines in Chapter 2 to have been evaluated in clinical studies. The evidence for acupuncture from one

RCT found no benefit, compared to no treatment, in terms of SCORAD and itch intensity measured on VAS. Assessment of the quality of evidence using GRADE was not able to be conducted, as the comparisons for these interventions were not considered to be critically important by the expert panel. There is insufficient evidence from the included studies to comment on the safety of this therapy.

Other CM therapies are used less frequently for atopic dermatitis than CHM and acupuncture therapies. One therapy was recommended in clinical practice guidelines and textbooks included in Chapter 2: *tuina* 推拿. However, no citations were identified in classical literature that described *tuina* 推拿, and no clinical studies specifically evaluated this technique. One study combined *tuina* 推拿 with CHM and moxibustion; however, as this study was a non-controlled study, we were unable to evaluate efficacy.

Acupuncture Therapies in Key Clinical Guidelines and Textbooks, Classical Literature and Clinical Studies

Some consistency was noted in the acupuncture therapies used for atopic dermatitis across the different types of evidence. Acupuncture is recommended in textbooks/guidelines included in Chapter 2 and has been evaluated in clinical studies (Table 9.4). It appears that it is more common to evaluate the efficacy of acupuncture used in combination with CHM (see Chapter 8), which is reflective of clinical practice. Acupuncture was infrequently used in classical literature, with only one citation describing its use for atopic dermatitis.

Other acupuncture-related interventions that have been recommended in textbooks and guidelines included in Chapter 2 were not evaluated alone in the included clinical studies and were seldom combined with other CM therapies. In fact, despite ear acupuncture and electroacupuncture being recommended by guidelines in Chapter 2, no studies were identified that were eligible for inclusion for review in Chapter 7. There is a need for rigorous studies that evaluate acupuncture therapies using validated outcomes relevant to atopic dermatitis.

Table 9.4. Summary of Acupuncture and Related Therapies

Intervention	Clinical Guidelines and Textbooks (Chapter 2)	Classical Literature (Chapter 3) (No. of Citations)	Clinical Studies in Chapter 7 (No. of Studies)			Combination Therapies (Chapter 8) (No. of Studies)
			RCTs	CCTs	Non-controlled Studies*	
Acupuncture	Yes	1	1	0	2	4
Moxibustion	Yes	0	0	0	0	1
Ear acupuncture	Yes	0	0	0	0	0
Electroacupuncture	Yes	0	0	0	0	0
Plum blossom needle therapy	Yes	0	0	0	0	1
Cupping	No	0	1	0	0	0

*Some studies used more than one intervention e.g. acupuncture plus moxibustion. These are counted separately in this table.

Abbreviations: RCTs, randomised controlled trials; CCTs, controlled clinical trials.

In addition to acupuncture, three other acupuncture interventions were included in Chapter 7. Acupressure, transcutaneous electrical nerve stimulation and cupping were used in RCTs and non-controlled studies. Findings from one RCT suggest acupressure may improve itch and lichenification. This intervention is worthy of further evaluation, as acupressure can be taught to patients for self-administration at home. If effective, this could provide a cost-effective treatment option for some patients.

While *tuina* 推拿 is considered an important intervention in the contemporary literature described in Chapter 2, there is insufficient evidence from the studies included in Chapter 7 to support its use in clinical practice. Two citations from the Qing dynasty described pricking the skin to withdraw blood. Chinese medicine practitioners should use their clinical judgment when considering these therapies for patients with atopic dermatitis.

A comparison of acupuncture points used across the different evidence types was conducted. Acupuncture points recommended in

Table 9.5.   Summary of Acupuncture Points

Intervention	Clinical Guidelines and Textbooks (Chapter 2)	Classical Literature (Chapter 3) (No. of Citations)	Clinical Studies in Chapter 7 (No. of Studies)			Combination Therapies (Chapter 8) (No. of Studies)
			RCTs	CCTs	Non-controlled Studies*	
LI11 *Quchi* 曲池	Yes	0	2	0	1	2
BL40 *Weizhong* 委中	Yes	0	0	0	0	0
SP10 *Xuehai* 血海	Yes	0	1	0	1	1
ST36 *Zusanli* 足三里	Yes	0	1	0	2	2
SP6 *Sanyinjiao* 三阴交	Yes	0	0	0	1	1
SP9 *Yinlingquan* 阴陵泉	Yes	0	0	0	1	1
GV14 *Dazhui* 大椎	Yes	0	0	0	1	1
BL13 *Feishu* 肺俞	Yes	0	0	0	0	0
CO14 Lung 肺	Yes	0	0	0	0	0
TG2p *Shenshangxian* (Adrenal gland) 肾上腺	Yes	0	0	0	0	0
CO18 *Neifenmi* (Endocrine) 内分泌	Yes	0	0	0	0	0
CO13 *Pi* (Spleen) 脾	Yes	0	0	0	0	0
TF4 *Shenmen* 神门	Yes	0	0	0	0	0

Note: Some studies used more than one intervention. These are counted separately in this table. Abbreviations: RCTs, randomised controlled trials; CCTs, controlled clinical trials.

textbooks and guidelines included in Chapter 2 and those used in two or more RCTs are described in Table 9.5. Several acupuncture points that are recommended in textbooks and guidelines have been used in included clinical studies. These are ST36 *Zusanli* 足三里 and LI11 *Quchi* 曲池 (used in five studies each), SP10 *Xuehai* 血海 (three studies), SP6 *Sanyinjiao* 三阴交 (two studies), SP9 *Yinlingquan* 阴陵泉 (two studies) and GV14 *Dazhui* 大椎 (two studies). These points address the two core concepts in atopic dermatitis: wind and Spleen deficiency with dampness. These points may be selected for patients with atopic dermatitis, in conjunction with points to address syndrome differentiation.

Limitations of Evidence

In collecting information for inclusion in this book, every effort was made to ensure accuracy of the content. The clinical guidelines and textbooks that describe CM syndromes and treatments in Chapter 2 were highly authoritative in the field of Chinese medicine. Despite this, it is possible that other textbooks and guidelines exist that may describe different syndromes and treatments. As such, the contents in Chapter 2 should not be considered the only syndromes and treatments for atopic dermatitis.

As described in Chapter 3, the *Zhong Hua Yi Dian* 中华医典 is a large collection of classical Chinese medicine texts,[10] and its digital format facilitates searching. The search of classical literature is limited by three factors: (1) the selected search terms; (2) the books included in the *Zhong Hua Yi Dian* 中华医典; and (3) the amount of information described in the identified citations. In relation to the first factor, search terms were selected based on consulting dermatology textbooks and clinical experts. As was highlighted in Chapter 3, other terms exist that may have been used for atopic dermatitis in classical Chinese language, although it is difficult to say definitively which terms were related to atopic dermatitis.

The majority of critical classical Chinese medicine books are included in the *Zhong Hua Yi Dian* 中华医典, but this collection does not include all books written from the pre-Tang dynasty to the modern era. References to atopic dermatitis included in different texts may provide a different perspective on the pathogenesis and treatment of atopic dermatitis. Criteria from previous research[11] were used to select citations that were possible cases of atopic dermatitis. It is possible that citations that provided insufficient information to permit a judgment of the likelihood of being atopic dermatitis were in fact related to atopic dermatitis. In conducting this analysis, decisions about eligibility had to be made based on the available information. Research using different search terms, searching a different collection of books and using different criteria to select citations may produce results different to those described in Chapter 3. A further limitation related to Chapter 3 is in the classical literature itself. Classical

Chinese language use and meaning have changed over time, thus it is possible that despite best efforts there are errors in the translated meanings of some phrases/citations.

Another limitation is that selection of search terms and the search strategies used to identify clinical evidence were designed to conduct a comprehensive search of relevant databases. Using different terms and different search parameters or selecting different eligibility criteria may alter the findings. Due to the sheer volume of records identified, errors may have occurred during classification of studies, resulting in potentially relevant studies being excluded. In addition, clinical studies that were selected for inclusion were those where the comparator was no treatment, placebo/sham or guideline-recommended treatments. We attempted to locate all relevant clinical guidelines to identify conventional medical management of atopic dermatitis, but this may not have been achieved. Differences in clinical practice guidelines were noted, and the comparators used in clinical studies may not be reflective of practice in any given geographical location.

Information from clinical studies related to patient demographics was extracted where available. This included information about the population under study (for example, participant age and severity of disease). Whilst conducting subgroup analysis according to participant demographics would have resulted in more direct evidence for specific patient groups, this was not able to be performed due to a lack of detail in many included studies. This was also the case in relation to CM syndrome differentiation. Over one-third of clinical studies described syndromes, yet only one reported outcome results according to the three syndromes seen. There is insufficient evidence from included studies to say which treatments would be most suitable for any given syndrome.

Lack of detail in study reports was noted for many studies. As a result the risk of bias assessment for some domains in RCTs was judged as unclear. This was particularly noted for risk of bias domains related to allocation concealment (how group allocation was concealed from patients and personnel) and selective outcome reporting (whether outcomes reported differed from those in a published protocol or clinical trial register). Of particular note, participants and personnel were not able to be blinded to group allocation in many studies due to the nature of the comparison. For example, where the intervention was a CHM decoction to be prepared by patients and the comparator was TCS, blinding of participants was not possible. Some studies attempted to blind participants and personnel through the use of a 'double dummy' design, but these were in the minority. In some cases, the lack of detail reduced our certainty in the results.

When considering the findings for all RCTs, practitioners should note that many studies compared CM interventions with antihistamines. Antihistamines are recommended in clinical practice guidelines as an adjuvant treatment in some guidelines[2,12] and as a first-line therapy in others.[13] Antihistamines may be helpful to reduce pruritus, but have not been shown to have any effect on atopic dermatitis scores.[2] Meta-analyses were conducted comparing CM interventions with pharmacotherapy, which may have included antihistamines, TCS and other guideline-recommended treatments. Subgroup analysis was conducted where possible according to comparator type, but due to the small number of studies, this was not always able to be performed. Thus the benefits of CM interventions against specific drug classes were not determined.

Many of the outcome measures used in atopic dermatitis are well known and have been validated in patients with atopic dermatitis. These outcomes were frequently used in clinical studies. Effective rate is an outcome often used in studies originating from China and provides a global assessment of the change in disease severity. The criteria for assessing the effective rate for a range of health conditions are described in CM clinical practice guidelines. Even so, many researchers develop their own criteria to categorise improvement. This creates a challenge when planning meta-analyses. Two highly authoritative and often used guidelines were selected as an outcome for evaluating evidence to reduce potential heterogeneity arising from different criteria used among studies. In doing so, it meant that the effective rate results for many studies were not analysed. Data from these studies may, or may not, alter the findings from this review. Furthermore, evaluation of results from clinical studies was conducted in aggregate, meaning that it was likely that the characteristics of clinical studies included in the meta-analysis were different. Clinical heterogeneity was anticipated, and the random effects model was used for statistical analysis to provide a more conservative estimate of the treatment effect.

Long-term control is important in atopic dermatitis to reduce the patient burden. The number of studies that reported recurrence was not small; however, differences in approaches used to assess recurrence prevented meta-analysis of all studies. For example, some studies assessed all participants for recurrence while others assessed only those who achieved a clinical improvement (based on effective rate) at the end of treatment. In the absence of a standard approach for measuring this outcome, difficulties are encountered when attempting to evaluate the potential benefit for CM interventions in achieving long-term control.

Frequency analysis was conducted to examine interventions identified in classical literature and those evaluated in clinical studies. As the volume of data in some cases was large, we have presented a selection of the most frequently used treatments, including CHM formulas and herbs, and acupuncture points. As such, some treatments which have been reported/examined less frequently may not appear unless their inclusion is noted in meta-analyses. Furthermore, when comparing herbs or acupuncture points used across the different types of evidence, one may not see instances reported across all sources, but this should not be taken to mean that consistency did not exist.

Implications for Practice

The clinical textbooks and guidelines included in Chapter 2 provide insight into the syndromes relevant to atopic dermatitis and guidance on selecting appropriate CM treatments for patients. The concepts described in syndromes in Chapter 2 are consistent with those reported in classical literature and in clinical studies. The classical literature in Chapter 3 provides historical context for CM management of atopic dermatitis. It should be noted that treatments described in this chapter may no longer be in use, and as such the content should not be taken as recommendations for clinical management.

Many of the syndromes described in clinical studies were similar to those described in clinical guidelines and textbooks, despite few studies evaluating clinical guideline-recommended CHM formulas or other interventions. This shows that the treatments in clinical studies were still addressing the underlying pathogenesis for people with atopic dermatitis. It remains unclear whether the other CM treatments that were not recommended in guidelines in Chapter 2 offer greater, lesser or equivalent benefit to treatments that were recommended in conventional medicine guidelines.

The results from RCTs provide the best evidence for the potential effects of CM treatments. Promising benefits were seen with oral, topical and the combination of oral plus topical CHM for some outcomes, but not others. Benefits were seen when CHM was used alone and when combined with guideline-recommended treatments. Many studies used investigator-developed formulas, and diversity was seen in the traditional formulas used in RCTs. This meant that it was not possible to conduct meta-analysis of individual formulas. As such, we are unable to provide evidence of the effects of specific formulas.

Herbs used in studies included in meta-analysis favouring CHM may provide some indication of which herbs have important actions for atopic dermatitis. Such herbs include *gan cao* 甘草, *bai zhu* 白术, *yi yi ren* 薏苡仁, *bai xian pi* 白鲜皮 and *fu ling* 茯苓 for oral use, and *huang bai* 黄柏 for topical use. Clinicians may wish to select formulas containing these herbs or consider using these herbs as modifications to existing formulas. Such an approach should also consider the patient's syndrome differentiation when formulating a treatment plan.

There was limited evidence for acupuncture therapies and other CM therapies. Two acupuncture points were used in three acupuncture therapy clinical studies: LI11 *Quchi* 曲池 and ST36 *Zusanli* 足三里. Both of these points were recommended in clinical guidelines in Chapter 2. The points are important for atopic dermatitis. Acupuncture point LI11 *Quchi* 曲池 clears heat, cools Blood, eliminates wind, drains damp and alleviates itching, while ST36 *Zusanli* 足三里 strengthens the Spleen, resolves dampness, tonifies *qi*, nourishes Blood and *yin*, and clears fire.[14] Clinicians may wish to consider other acupuncture points based on syndrome differentiation when using acupuncture-related interventions.

Across all clinical evidence chapters, the most useful evidence for the effects of CM interventions for atopic dermatitis can be found in the GRADE assessments. These assessments answer clinically important questions, where CM interventions are compared to pharmacotherapy directly targeting atopic dermatitis and its relevant mechanisms i.e., TCS and TCIs. Unfortunately, few studies made such comparisons, and the overall quality of the evidence was low. This means we are not certain that these results reflect the true treatment effect, and further research is highly likely to change the findings.

Many patients seek complementary and alternative medicine with the belief that these are safe to use.[15,16] This is the case in atopic dermatitis, where long-term use of some treatments, such as TCS, is associated with side effects. Chinese medicine interventions are not without side effects and this should be considered when selecting treatments for patients. Mild adverse events with oral CHM were seen and tended to be gastrointestinal in nature. Fewer adverse events were reported with topical CHM than with pharmacotherapy, and these were gastrointestinal or dermatological in nature. Few studies of acupuncture and other CM therapies reported on adverse events and there remains insufficient evidence for their safety. Patients should also be advised of the potential risks with treatment, and collaboratively a choice can be made about the most appropriate treatment for each individual.

Implications for Research

The growing shift towards evidence-based practice demands high-quality studies to inform clinical decision making. The number of studies evaluating CM interventions for atopic dermatitis is growing, yet there is more work to be done. Further research is needed to confirm the promising effects seen in the included studies and to continue to examine possible interventions. Future trials should be rigorous, use validated outcomes and be registered in clinical trial registers to ensure transparency in trial reporting. Blinding remains an issue in studies where CM interventions are compared with pharmacotherapy or phototherapy. Some studies included in Chapter 5 used a placebo CHM to ensure blinding of participants. Such an approach will further reduce potential bias due to lack of participants blinding. Few of the included studies provided the details required by Consolidated Standards of Reporting Trials (CONSORT)[17] and extensions for herbal medicine,[18] acupuncture[19] and moxibustion.[20] Adherence to these reporting requirements will increase transparency in clinical studies and allow for study replication.

Many validated outcomes exist for atopic dermatitis, and the Harmonising Outcome Measures for Eczema (HOME) consensus have recommended core outcome domains include signs, symptoms, quality of life and long-term control.[21] Consensus has been reached that the Eczema Area Severity Index (EASI)[22] be used for clinician-reported signs and Patient-oriented Eczema Measure (POEM)[23] be used for patient-reported symptoms. Consensus is yet to be reached on the other domains. These outcomes were infrequently used in the included clinical studies despite being available for many years. Inclusion of EASI and POEM in future clinical trial designs will reduce variation in outcome measures and will permit pooling of data to estimate the treatment effect.

In the absence of a core instrument for assessing quality of life, the DLQI[24] (and variants for children and infants) remains a popular tool. Several included studies used the adult and child versions, and results were presented in aggregate. This approach has been criticised,[25] as these versions include questions specific to each age group and scoring characteristics are different. Researchers who intend to use age-specific versions of this outcome tool are encouraged to report the results of each version separately. Long-term control remains a key concern for both clinicians and patients. Consensus on a core outcome for assessing recurrence will provide researchers with a clearer method, will reduce variation and will increase the ability to pool results from different studies.

The herbs used in multiple studies in positive meta-analysis (Chapter 5) provide promising avenues for drug discovery. Some of these herbs were selected for review of experimental studies. Evidence suggests some herbs exhibit anti-allergic, antipruritic, anti-inflammatory, and immunomodulatory mechanisms relevant to atopic dermatitis. When used in clinical studies, authentication of CHM formulas and herb ingredients should be undertaken and the process used should be described. Efforts should be made to quantify the amount of active constituents.

Several of the treatments recommended by clinical textbooks and guidelines included in Chapter 2 appear to lack evidence of their effect. For example, no studies were included that evaluated moxibustion, ear acupuncture, electroacupuncture, plum blossom needling or *tuina* 推拿. Furthermore, several of the CHM formulas were not evaluated in clinical studies. It is important for research to be conducted on these interventions so clinicians can be more confident there is evidence to support their use.

References

1. Katayama I, Kohno Y, Akiyama K, *et al.* (2014) Japanese guideline for atopic dermatitis 2014. *Allergol Int* **63**(3): 377–398.
2. Wollenberg A, Oranje A, Deleuran M, *et al.* (2016) ETFAD/EADV Eczema Task Force 2015 position paper on diagnosis and treatment of atopic dermatitis in adult and paediatric patients. *J Eur Acad Dermatol Venereol* **30**(5): 729–747.
3. Eichenfield LF, Tom WL, Berger TG, *et al.* (2014) Guidelines of care for the management of atopic dermatitis: Section 2. Management and treatment of atopic dermatitis with topical therapies. *J Am Acad Dermatol* **71**(1): 116–132.
4. Sidbury R, Davis DM, Cohen DE, *et al.* (2014) Guidelines of care for the management of atopic dermatitis: Section 3. Management and treatment with phototherapy and systemic agents. *J Am Acad Dermatol* **71**(2): 327–349.

5. Katayama I, Aihara M, Ohya Y, *et al.* (2017) Japanese guidelines for atopic dermatitis 2017. *Allergol Int* **66**(2): 230–247.

6. (1993) Severity scoring of atopic dermatitis: The SCORAD index. Consensus report of the European Task Force on Atopic Dermatitis. *Dermatology* **186:** 23–31.

7. Bensky D, Clavey S, Stoger E. (2004) *Chinese Herbal Medicine Materia Medica*, 3rd ed. Eastland Press, Inc., Seattle, US.

8. Coyle M, Liang H, Wang K, *et al.* (2018) In: Xue C, Lu C (eds.), *Herpes Zoster and Post-herpetic Neuralgia, Volume 6.* World Scientific Publishing Co. Pte. Ltd., New Jersey, US.

9. Coyle M, Yu J, Di Y, *et al.* (2017) In: Xue C, Lu C (eds.), *Chronic Urticaria, Volume 3.* World Scientific Publishing Co. Pte. Ltd., New Jersey, US.

10. May B, Lu Y, Lu C, *et al.* (2013) Systematic assessment of the representativeness of published collections of the traditional literature on Chinese medicine. *J Altern Complement Med* **19**: 403–409.

11. 黄楚君, 蔡坚雄, 刘炽, 黄咏菁, 吴大嵘, 陈达灿. (2011) 特应性皮炎古籍文献的内容评析. 时珍国医国药 **22**(6): 1492–1494.

12. Saeki H, Nakahara T, Tanaka A, *et al.* (2016) Clinical practice guidelines for the management of atopic dermatitis 2016. *J Dermatol* **43**(10): 1117–1145.

13. Schneider L, Tilles S, Lio P, *et al.* (2013) Atopic dermatitis: A practice parameter update 2012. *J Allergy Clin Immunol* **131**(2): 295–299. e1–e27.

14. Deadman P, Al-Khafaji M, Baker K. (2000) *A Manual of Acupuncture.* Journal of Chinese Medicine Publications, East Sussex, UK.

15. Chan TY, Critchley JA. (1996) Usage and adverse effects of Chinese herbal medicines. *Hum Exp Toxicol* **15**(1): 5–12.

16. George J, Ioannides-Demos LL, Santamaria NM, *et al.* (2004) Use of complementary and alternative medicines by patients with chronic obstructive pulmonary disease. *Med J Aust* **181**(5): 248–251.

17. Schulz KF, Altman DG, Moher D. (2010) CONSORT 2010 statement: Updated guidelines for reporting parallel group randomised trials. *PLoS Med* **7**(3): e1000251.

18. Gagnier JJ, Boon H, Rochon P, *et al.* (2006) Reporting randomized, controlled trials of herbal interventions: An elaborated CONSORT statement. *Ann Intern Med* **144**(5): 364–367.

19. MacPherson H, Altman DG, Hammerschlag R, *et al.* (2010) Revised standards for reporting interventions in clinical trials of acupuncture

(STRICTA): Extending the consort statement. *J Evid Based Med* **3**(3): 140–155.

20. Cheng CW, Fu SF, Zhou QH, *et al.* (2013) Extending the CONSORT statement to moxibustion. *J Integr Med* **11**(1): 54–63.

21. Chalmers JR, Simpson E, Apfelbacher CJ, *et al.* (2016) Report from the fourth international consensus meeting to harmonize core outcome measures for atopic eczema/dermatitis clinical trials (HOME initiative). *Br J Dermatol* **175**(1): 69–79.

22. Tofte S, Graeber M, Cherill R, *et al.* (1998) Eczema area and severity index (EASI): A new tool to evaluate atopic dermatitis. *J Eur Acad Dermatol Venereol* **11**: S197.

23. Charman CR, Venn AJ, Williams HC. (2004) The patient-oriented eczema measure: Development and initial validation of a new tool for measuring atopic eczema severity from the patients' perspective. *Arch Dermatol* **140**(12): 1513–1519.

24. Finlay A, Khan G. (1994) Dermatology Life Quality Index (DLQI): A simple practical measure for routine clinical use. *Clin Exp Dermatol* **19**(3): 210–216.

25. Finlay AY, Basra MKA. (2012) DLQI and CDLQI scores should not be combined. *Br J Dermatol* **167**(2): 453–454.

Glossary

Glossary of Terms	Acronym	Definition	Reference
95% Confidence Interval	95% CI	A measure of the uncertainty around the main finding of a statistical analysis. Estimates of unknown quantities, such as the odds ratio comparing an experimental intervention with a control, are usually presented as a point estimate and a 95% confidence interval. This means that if someone were to keep repeating a study in other samples from the same population, 95% of the confidence intervals from those studies would contain the true value of the unknown quantity. Alternatives to 95%, such as 90% and 99% confidence intervals, are sometimes used. Wider intervals indicate lower precision; narrow intervals, greater precision.	https://training.cochrane.org/handbook
Acupressure	—	Application of pressure on acupuncture points.	—
Acupuncture	—	The insertion of needles into humans or animals for remedial purposes.	World Health Organisation. (2007) WHO International Standard Terminologies of Traditional Medicine in the Western Pacific Region.
Allied and Complementary Medicine Database	AMED	Alternative medicine bibliographic database.	www.ebsco.com/products/research-databases/allied-and-complementary-medicine-database-amed

(Continued)

(*Continued*)

Glossary of Terms	Acronym	Definition	Reference
Australian New Zealand Clinical Trial Registry	ANZCTR	Clinical trial registry based in Australia.	www.anzctr.org.au/
Children's Dermatology Life Quality Index	CDLQI	Scale for measuring the impact of atopic dermatitis in children, developed from the DLQI.	Lewis-Jones MS, Finlay AY. (1995) The Children's Dermatology Life Quality Index (CDLQI): Initial validation and practical use. *Br J Dermatol* **132**(6): 942–949.
China National Knowledge Infrastructure	CNKI	Chinese language bibliographic database.	www.cnki.net
Chinese Biomedical Literature Database	CBM	Chinese language bibliographic database.	www.imicams.ac.cn
Chinese Clinical Trial Registry	ChiCTR	Chinese clinical trial registry.	http://www.chictr.org.cn/
Chinese herbal medicine	CHM	—	—
Chinese medicine	CM	—	—
Chongqing VIP Information Company	CQVIP	Chinese language bibliographic database.	www.cqvip.com
ClinicalTrials.gov	—	Clinical trial registry based in the United States.	https://clinicaltrials.gov/
Cochrane Central Register of Controlled Trials	CENTRAL	Bibliographic database that provides a highly concentrated source of reports of controlled trials.	https://community.cochrane.org/editorial-and-publishing-policy-resource/overview-cochrane-library-and-related-content/databases-included-cochrane-library/cochrane-central-register-controlled-trials-central
Combination therapies	—	Two or more Chinese medicines from different therapy groups (e.g. Chinese herbal medicine, acupuncture therapies or other Chinese medicine therapies) administered together.	—
Controlled clinical trials	CCT	A study in which people are allocated to different interventions using methods that are not random.	https://training.cochrane.org/handbook

(*Continued*)

(Continued)

Glossary of Terms	Acronym	Definition	Reference
Convention on International Trade in Endangered Species of Wild Fauna and Flora	CITES	International convention aimed at preventing, or regulating, trade in threatened and endangered species of plants and animals.	https://www.cites.org/eng/disc/text.php
Cumulative Index of Nursing and Allied Health Literature	CINAHL	Bibliographic database.	https://www.ebscohost.com/nursing/products/cinahl-databases
Cupping therapy	—	Suction by using a vacuumised cup or jar.	World Health Organisation. (2007) WHO International Standard Terminologies of Traditional Medicine in the Western Pacific Region.
Eczema Area and Severity Index	EASI	Tool for assessing severity of eczema/atopic dermatitis (clinical signs).	Tofte S, Graeber M, Cherill R, *et al.* (1998) Eczema area and severity index (EASI): A new tool to evaluate atopic dermatitis. *J Eur Acad Dermatol Venereol* **11**: S197.
Dermatology Life Quality Index	DLQI	Scale for measuring the impact of atopic dermatitis.	Finlay A, Khan G. (1994) Dermatology Life Quality Index (DLQI): A simple practical measure for routine clinical use. *Clin Exp Dermatol* **19**(3): 210–216.
Effect size	—	A generic term for the estimate of the effect of a treatment for a study.	http://handbook.cochrane.org/
Effective rate	ER	A measure of the proportion of participants who achieved an improvement, as outlined in the methods for evaluating clinical evidence section.	—
Electroacupuncture	—	Electric stimulation of the needle following insertion.	World Health Organisation. (2007) WHO International Standard Terminologies of Traditional Medicine in the Western Pacific Region.
EU Clinical Trials Register	EU-CTR	European Clinical Trial Registry.	https://www.clinicaltrialsregister.eu
Excerpta Medica dataBASE	Embase	Bibliographic database.	http://www.elsevier.com/solutions/embase

(Continued)

(Continued)

Glossary of Terms	Acronym	Definition	Reference
Grading of Recommendations Assessment, Development and Evaluation	GRADE	Approach used to grade quality of evidence and strength of recommendations.	http://www.gradeworkinggroup.org/
Health-related quality of life	HRQoL	A conceptual or operational measurement that is commonly used in a health care setting as a means to assess the impact of a disease on a person.	(2010) *Brooker C. Mosby's Dictionary of Medicine, Nursing and Health Professions.* Elsevier, United Kingdom.
Heterogeneity	—	Used in a general sense to describe the variation in, or diversity of, participants, interventions and measurement of outcomes across a set of studies, or the variation in internal validity of those studies. Used specifically, as statistical heterogeneity, to describe the degree of variation in the effect estimates from a set of studies. Also used to indicate the presence of variability among studies beyond the amount expected due solely to the play of chance.	https://training.cochrane.org/handbook
Harmonising Outcome Measures for Eczema	HOME	Consensus group formed to identify a core set of outcome measures for clinical trials of eczema.	Chalmers JR, Simpson E, Apfelbacher CJ, *et al.* (2016) Report from the fourth international consensus meeting to harmonize core outcome measures for atopic eczema/dermatitis clinical trials (HOME initiative). *Br J Dermatol* **175**(1): 69–79.
Homogeneity	—	Used in a general sense to mean that the participants, interventions and measurement of outcomes are similar across a set of studies. Used specifically to describe the effect estimates from a set of studies where they do not vary more than would be expected by chance.	https://training.cochrane.org/handbook

(Continued)

Glossary

(*Continued*)

Glossary of Terms	Acronym	Definition	Reference
I^2	—	A measure of study heterogeneity; indicates the percentage of variance in a meta-analysis.	https://training.cochrane.org/handbook
Integrative medicine	IM	Chinese herbal medicine combined with pharmacotherapy or other conventional therapy.	—
Mean difference	MD	In meta-analysis, a method used to combine measures on continuous scales, where the mean, standard deviation and sample size in each group are known. The weight given to the difference in means from each study (e.g. how much influence each study has on the overall results of the meta-analysis) is determined by the precision of its estimate of effect; mathematically this is equal to the inverse of the variance. This method assumes that all of the trials have measured the outcome on the same scale.	https://training.cochrane.org/handbook
Meta-analysis	—	The use of statistical techniques in a systematic review to integrate the results of included studies. Sometimes misused as a synonym for systematic reviews, where the review includes a meta-analysis.	https://training.cochrane.org/handbook
Moxibustion	—	A therapeutic procedure involving ignited material (usually moxa) to apply heat to certain points or areas of the body surface for managing disease.	World Health Organisation. (2007) WHO International Standard Terminologies of Traditional Medicine in the Western Pacific Region.
Non-controlled studies	—	Observations made on individuals, usually receiving the same intervention, before and after an intervention but with no control group.	https://training.cochrane.org/handbook

(*Continued*)

(Continued)

Glossary of Terms	Acronym	Definition	Reference
Other Chinese medicine therapies	—	Other Chinese medicine therapies include all traditional therapies except Chinese herbal medicine and acupuncture/moxibustion, such as *tai chi* 太極, *qi gong* 气功, *tuina* 推拿 and cupping.	—
Patient-oriented Eczema Measure	POEM	Tool for assessing eczema/atopic dermatitis symptoms.	Charman CR, Venn AJ, Williams HC. (2004) The patient-oriented eczema measure: Development and initial validation of a new tool for measuring atopic eczema severity from the patients' perspective. *Arch Dermatol* **140**(12): 1513–1519.
PubMed	PubMed	Bibliographic database.	http://www.ncbi.nlm.nih.gov/pubmed
Randomised controlled trial	RCT	Clinical trial that uses a random method to allocate participants to treatment and control groups.	—
Risk of bias	—	Assessment of clinical trials to indicate if the results may overestimate or underestimate the true effect because of bias in study design or reporting.	http://handbook.cochrane.org/
Risk ratio	RR	The ratio of risks in two groups. In intervention studies, it is the ratio of the risk in the intervention group to the risk in the control group. A risk ratio of 1 indicates no difference between comparison groups. For undesirable outcomes, a risk ratio that is less than 1 indicates that the intervention was effective in reducing the risk of that outcome.	https://training.cochrane.org/handbook

(Continued)

(Continued)

Glossary of Terms	Acronym	Definition	Reference
Six Area, Six Signs Atopic Dermatitis	SASSAD	Scale for measuring clinical signs of atopic dermatitis.	Berth-Jones J. (1996) Six area, six-sign atopic dermatitis (SASSAD) severity score: A simple system for monitoring disease activity in atopic dermatitis. *Br J Dermatol* **135**(Suppl 48): 25–30.
SCOring Atopic Dermatitis Index	SCORAD	Scale for assessing severity of atopic dermatitis.	(1993) Severity scoring of atopic dermatitis: The SCORAD index. Consensus Report of the European Task Force on Atopic Dermatitis. *Dermatology* **186**: 23–31.
Standardised mean difference	SMD	In meta-analysis, a method used to combine results for continuous scales which measure the same outcome, but for which these outcomes were measured in different ways (e.g. with different scales). The results of studies are standardised to a uniform scale to allow data to be combined.	https://training.cochrane.org/handbook
Summary of findings	SoF	Presentation of results and rating the quality of evidence based on the GRADE approach.	http://www.gradeworkinggroup.org/
Three-item Severity scale	TIS	Short scale for measuring disease severity in clinical practice.	Wolkerstorfer A, de Waard van der Spek FB, Glazenburg EJ, *et al.* (1999) Scoring the severity of atopic dermatitis: Three-item severity score as a rough system for daily practice and as a pre-screening tool for studies. *Acta Derm Venereol* **79**(5): 356–359.
Transcutaneous electrical nerve stimulation	TENS	Application of transdermal electrical current to acupuncture points via conducting pads.	—
Topical corticosteroid	TCS	Topical treatment for atopic dermatitis.	—
Topical calcineurin inhibitor	TCI	Topical treatment for atopic dermatitis.	—

(Continued)

(Continued)

Glossary of Terms	Acronym	Definition	Reference
Tuina 推拿	—	Chinese massage: rubbing, kneading or percussion of the soft tissues and joints of the body with the hands, usually performed by one person on another, especially to relieve tension or pain.	World Health Organisation (2007) WHO International Standard Terminologies of Traditional Medicine in the Western Pacific Region.
Wanfang database	Wanfang	Chinese language bibliographic database.	www.wanfangdata.com
World Health Organisation	WHO	WHO is the directing and coordinating authority for health within the United Nations system. It is responsible for providing leadership on global health matters, shaping the health research agenda, setting norms and standards, articulating evidence-based policy options, providing technical support to countries and monitoring and assessing health trends.	http://www.who.int/about/en/
Zhong Hua Yi Dian 中华医典	ZHYD	The *Zhong Hua Yi Dian* (ZHYD) (*Encyclopaedia of Traditional Chinese Medicine*) is a comprehensive series of electronic books on compact disk. The collection was put together by the Hunan Electronic and Audio-Visual Publishing House. It is the largest collection of Chinese electronic books and includes the major Chinese ancient works, many of which are from rare manuscripts and are the only existing copies. These books cover the period from ancient times up to the period of the Republic of China (1911–1948).	Hu R, ed. (2000) *Zhong Hua Yi Dian (Encyclopaedia of Traditional Chinese Medicine)*, 4th ed. Hunan Electronic and Audio-Visual Publishing House, Chengsha.

(Continued)

(Continued)

Glossary of Terms	Acronym	Definition	Reference
Zhong Yi Fang Ji Da Ci Dian 中医方剂大辞典	ZYFJDCD	Compendium of Chinese herbal formulas with over 96,592 entries derived from classical Chinese books. The Nanjing Chinese Medicine Institute compiled the ZYFJDCD and first published it in 1993.	Peng HR, ed. (1994) *Zhong Yi Fang Ji Da Ci Dian (Great Compendium of Chinese Medical Formulas)*. People's Medical Publishing House, Beijing.

Index

Evidence-based Clinical Chinese Medicine

Print ISSN: 2529-7562
Online ISSN: 2529-7554

Series Co Editors-in-Chief

Charlie Changli Xue *(RMIT University, Australia)*
Chuanjian Lu *(Guangdong Provincial Hospital of Chinese Medicine, China)*

Published

More information on this series can also be found at https://www.worldscientific.com/series/ebccm